THE DOCTOR'S GUIDE TO CRITICAL APPRAISAL

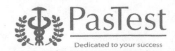

PasTest
Dedicated to your success

THE DOCTOR'S GUIDE TO CRITICAL APPRAISAL

Dr Narinder Kaur Gosall
BSc (Hons) PhD

Clinical Effectiveness Consultant
Pfizer Limited

Dr Gurpal Singh Gosall
MA MB BChir MRCPsych

Consultant General Adult Psychiatrist
Royal Blackburn Hospital, Lancashire

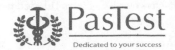

PasTest
Dedicated to your success

© 2006 PasTest Ltd

Egerton Court
Parkgate Estate
Knutsford
Cheshire WA16 8DX

Telephone: 01565 752000

First edition 2006

ISBN: 1 905635028
ISBN: 978 1 905635023

A catalogue record for this book is available from the British Library.

PasTest Revision Books and Intensive Courses

PasTest has been established in the field of postgraduate medical education since 1972, providing revision books and intensive study courses for doctors preparing for their professional examinations.

Books and courses are available for the following specialties:

MRCGP, MRCP Parts 1 and 2, MRCPCH Parts 1 and 2, MRCPsych, MRCS, MRCOG Parts 1 and 2, DRCOG, DCH, FRCA, PLAB Parts 1 and 2, Dental Students, Dentists and Dental Nurses.

For further details contact:

PasTest, Freepost, Knutsford, Cheshire WA16 7BR

Tel: 01565 752000   Fax: 01565 650264

www.pastest.co.uk   enquires@pastest.co.uk

Text prepared by Carnegie Book Production, Lancaster
Printed by MPG Books Ltd, Bodmin, Cornwall

CONTENTS

Dedicated to our baby son,
Dilip.

ABOUT THE AUTHORS

Dr Narinder Kaur Gosall BSc (Hons) PhD
Clinical Effectiveness Consultant, Pfizer Limited

Narinder Gosall studied in Liverpool and gained a PhD in neuropathology after investigating the role of the phrenic nerve in sudden infant death syndrome and intrauterine growth retardation. After working as a university lecturer, she joined the pharmaceutical industry and currently works as a Clinical Effectiveness Consultant for Pfizer Limited. She has extensive experience in teaching critical appraisal skills to doctors and has written more than 20 scientific publications.

Dr Gurpal Singh Gosall MA MB BChir MRCPsych
Consultant General Adult Psychiatrist, Royal Blackburn Hospital, Lancashire

Gurpal Gosall studied medicine at the University of Cambridge and Guy's and St Thomas's Hospitals, London. He worked as a Senior House Officer in Psychiatry in Leeds before working as a Specialist Registrar in the Manchester rotation. He now works as a Consultant Psychiatrist in Lancashire Care NHS Trust. He has had a long-standing interest in teaching and runs a popular website for psychiatrists, the Superego Cafe.

INTRODUCTION

One of the attractions of a career in medicine is that it is forever advancing. Hardly a day goes by without a new discovery about a disease process or an exciting innovation in the management of an illness. This book aims to help doctors who want to practice medicine at the leading edge. It is not enough simply to read the latest journal articles. Doctors need to examine critically the research laid before them and decide which evidence to take to the bedside. They need to lead their teams to higher standards of patient care based on robust evidence about what works and what doesn't work.

The skill of evaluating research is so valuable that there is no room for academic snobbery. We hope that this book is a refreshing change to the reader, explaining the principles of critical appraisal in an easy-to-read format. We have tried to make the subject appear as simple as possible – because it is simple. If, after reading this book, the reader is better able to evaluate the next journal article he or she reads, we will have done our job. Enjoy.

NKG, GSG

INTRODUCING CRITICAL APPRAISAL

Scenario 1

Dr Jones was annoyed. Six months ago, he was given a clinical paper by a pharmaceutical sales representative about a new treatment for high blood pressure. The results of the trial were certainly impressive. On the basis of the evidence presented, he prescribed the new tablet to all his hypertensive patients. Instead of the expected finding that four out of every five patients would lower their blood pressure, only one out of every ten of his patients improved. He decided to present the article in the hospital journal club, as he himself couldn't see where in the study the mistake lay. He then hoped to confront the sales representative for wasting his time and the hospital's money.

Every year, thousands of clinical papers are published in the medical press. The vast range of topics reflect the complexity of the human body, with studies all fighting for our attention. Separating the 'wheat from the chaff' is a daunting task for doctors, such that many rely on others for expert guidance.

In 1972, the publication of Archie Cochrane's *Effectiveness and Efficiency: Random Reflections on Health Services*[1] made doctors realise how unaware they were about the effects of health care. Archie Cochrane, a British epidemiologist, went on to set up the Cochrane Collaboration in 1992. It is now an international organisation, committed to producing and disseminating systematic reviews of health-care interventions. Bodies such as the Cochrane Collaboration have made the lives of doctors much easier, but the skill of evaluating evidence should be in the arsenal of every doctor.

Evidence-based medicine

Evidence-based medicine is the phrase used to describe the process of practising medicine based on a combination of the best available research evidence, our clinical expertise and patient values. As such, evidence-based medicine has had a tremendous impact on improving health-care outcomes since its widespread adoption in the early 1990s.

The most widely quoted definition of evidence-based medicine is that it is *'the conscientious, explicit and judicious use of current best evidence in making decisions about the care of the individual patient'*[2]. The practice of evidence-based medicine comprises 5 steps, shown in **Table 1**.

1 Cochrane AL. *Effectiveness and efficiency: random reflections on health services*. London, Royal Society of Medicine Press, 1999.
2 Sackett DL, Richardson WS, Rosenberg W, Haynes RB. *Evidence based medicine: how to practice and teach evidence based medicine*. London, Churchill Livingstone, 1997.

EVIDENCE BASED MEDICINE – THE FIVE STEPS		
1	Question	Formulate a precise, structured clinical question about an aspect of patient management.
2	Evidence	Search for the best evidence with which to answer the question.
3	Critical Appraisal	Evaluate the evidence, critically appraising the evidence for its validity, impact and applicability.
4	Application	Apply the results to clinical practice, integrating the critical appraisal with clinical expertise and with patients' circumstances.
5	Implementation and Monitoring	Implement and monitor this whole process, evaluating the effectiveness and efficacy of the whole process and identify ways to improve them both for the future.

Table 1 Evidence-based medicine – the five steps

Evidenced-based medicine begins with the formulation of a clinical question, such as *'what is the best treatment for carpal tunnel syndrome?'* This is followed by a search of the medical literature, looking for answers to the question. The evidence gathered is appraised and the results are applied to our patients. The final step, which is often overlooked, is to monitor any changes and repeat the process.

Critical appraisal

In the process of evidence-based medicine, why do we need a step on critical appraisal? Why not take all results at face value and apply all the findings to clinical practice? The first reason is that there may be conflicting conclusions drawn from different studies. Secondly, real-life medicine rarely follows the restrictive environments in which clinical trials take place. To apply, implement and monitor evidence, we need to ensure that the evidence we are looking at can be translated into our own clinical environments.

Critical appraisal is just one step in the process of evidence-based medicine, allowing doctors to assess the research found and decide which research will have a clinically significant impact on their patients. Critical appraisal allows doctors to exclude research that is too poorly designed to inform medical practice. By itself, critical appraisal does not lead to improved outcomes. It is only when the conclusions drawn from critically appraised studies are applied to everyday practice and monitored that the outcomes for patients improve.

Critical appraisal assesses the validity of the research and statistical techniques used in studies, and generates clinically useful information from them. It seeks to answer two major questions:

> Does the research have **internal validity**: to what extent do the results from the study reflect the true results by taking into consideration the study design and methodology?

> Does the research have **external validity**: to what extent can the results from the study be generalised to a wider population?

As with most subjects in medicine, it is not possible to learn about critical appraisal without coming across jargon. Wherever we start, we will come across words and phrases we do not understand. In this book, we try to explain critical appraisal in a logical and easy-to-remember way. Anything unfamiliar will be explained in due course.

Efficacy and effectiveness

Two words that are useful to define now are 'efficacy' and 'effectiveness'. They are sometimes used interchangeably, but they have different meanings and consequences in the context of evidence-based medicine.

Efficacy describes the impact of interventions under optimal (trial) conditions.

Effectiveness is a different but related concept, describing whether the interventions have the intended or expected effect under ordinary (clinical) circumstances.

Efficacy shows that internal validity is present. Effectiveness shows that external validity (generalisability) is present.

The contrast between efficacy and effectiveness studies was first highlighted 30 years ago by Schwartz and Lellouch[3]. Efficacy studies usually have the aim of seeking regulatory approval for licensing. The interventions in such studies tend to be strictly controlled and compared with placebo interventions. The people taking part in such studies tend to be a selective 'eligible' population. In contrast, effectiveness studies tend to be undertaken for formulary approval. Dosing regimens tend to be more flexible and compared with interventions already being used. Almost anyone is eligible to enter such trials.

It is not always easy and straightforward to translate the results from clinical trials (efficacy data) to uncontrolled clinical settings (effectiveness data). There are many factors which mean that results achieved in everyday practice do not always mirror an intervention's published efficacy data. The efficacy of an intervention is nearly always more impressive than its effectiveness.

Scenario 1 revisited

The journal club audience unanimously agreed that the double-blind randomised controlled trial was conducted to a high standard. The methodology, the analysis of the results and the conclusions drawn could not be criticised. When Dr Jones queried why his results were so different, the chairman of the journal club commented, "My colleague needs to understand the difference between efficacy data and his effectiveness data. I assume his outpatient clinic and follow-up arrangements are not run to the exacting standards of a major international trial! May I suggest that, before criticizing the work of others, he should perhaps read a book on critical appraisal?"

[3] Schwartz D, Lellouch J. Explanatory and pragmatic attitudes in therapeutical trials. *Journal of Chronic Diseases*, 1967, 20, 637–48.

SECTION A
FIRST IMPRESSIONS

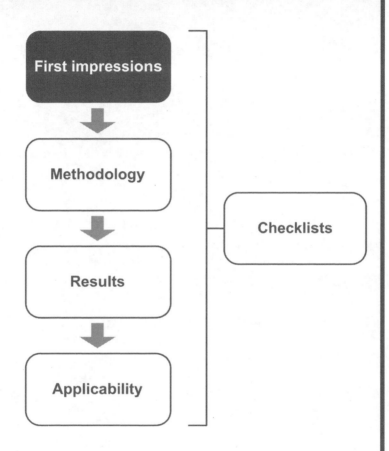

First impressions

Methodology

Results

Applicability

Checklists

THE JOURNAL

Not all journals are equal. Some journals are more prestigious than others. There may be many reasons for such prestige, including a long history in publishing, affiliation with an important medical organisation or a reputation for publishing important research. It is important to know in which journal an article was published – but remember, poor articles are published in even the best journals, and *vice versa*.

Peer-reviewed journals

A peer-reviewed journal is a publication that requires each submitted article to be independently examined by a panel of experts who are non-editorial staff of the journal. To be considered for publication, articles need to be approved by the majority of peers. The process is usually anonymous, with the authors not knowing the identities of the peer reviewers. In double-blind peer review, neither the author nor the reviewers know each others' identities. Anonymity aids the feedback process.

The peer review process forces authors to meet certain standards laid down by researchers and experts in that field. Peer review makes it more likely that mistakes or flaws in research are detected before publication. As a result of this quality assurance, **peer-reviewed journals are regarded in greater esteem than non-peer-reviewed journals**.

There are disadvantages to the peer review process. First, it adds a delay between the submission of an article and its publication. Secondly, the peer reviewers may guess the identity of the author(s), particularly in small specialised fields, impairing the objectivity of their assessments. Thirdly, revolutionary or unpopular conclusions may face opposition within the peer review process, leading to preservation of the *status quo*.

Journal impact factor

A **journal impact factor** provides a means of evaluating or comparing the performance of a journal relative to others in the same field. It ranks a journal's importance by the number of times articles within that journal are cited by others. A higher frequency of citation implies that the journal is found to be useful to others, suggesting that the research published in the journal is valuable. Impact factors are calculated annually by the Institute for Scientific Information and published in the Journal Citation Report.

The journal impact factor[4] is a measure of the frequency with which the average article in a journal has been cited in a particular year.

The **impact factor** is the number of citations in the current year to articles published in the two previous years, divided by the total number of articles published in the two previous years.

The **immediacy index** is another way of evaluating journals from the Institute for Scientific Information. It measures how often articles published in a journal are cited within the same year. This is useful for comparing journals specialising in cutting-edge research.

[4] *Journal citation report (JCR)*. Philadelphia, USA, Thomson Institute for Scientific Information, 2005. JCR provides quantitative tools for ranking, evaluating, categorising and comparing journals.

ORGANISATION OF THE ARTICLE

The majority of published articles follow a similar structure.

Title of the article: this should be concise and informative, but sometimes an attention-grabbing title is used to attract readers to an otherwise dull paper.

Author(s): this should allow you to see if the authors have the appropriate academic and professional qualifications and experience. The institutions at which the authors work may also be listed and may increase the credibility of the project if they have a good reputation for research in this field.

Abstract: this summarises the research paper, briefly describing the reasons for the research, the methodology, the overall findings and the conclusions made. Reading the abstract is a quick way of getting to know the article, but the brevity of the information given means that it is unlikely to reveal the strengths and weaknesses of the research. If the abstract is of interest to you, you must go on to read the rest of the article. Never rely on an abstract alone to inform your medical practice!

Introduction: this explains what the research is about and why the study was carried out. A good introduction will include references to previous work related to this subject matter and describe the importance and limitations of what is already known.

Method: this gives detailed information about how the study was actually carried out. Specific information is given on the study design, the population of interest, how the sample of the population was selected, the interventions offered and which outcomes were measured and how they were measured.

Results: this shows what happened to the individuals studied. It may include raw data and explain the statistical tests used to analyse the data. The results may be portrayed in tables, diagrams and graphs.

Conclusion / discussion: this discusses the results in the context of what is already known about the subject area and the clinical relevance of what has been found. It may include a discussion on the limitations of the research and suggestions on further research.

Conflicting interests / funding: articles should be published on their scientific merit. A conflicting interest is any factor that interferes with the objectivity of research findings. Conflicting interests can be held by anyone involved in the research project, from the formulation of a research proposal through to its publication, including authors, their employers, sponsoring organisation, journal editors and peer reviewers. Conflicting interests can be financial (eg research grants, honoraria for speaking at meetings), professional (eg member of organisational body) or personal (eg relationship with the journal's editor). Ideally, authors should disclose conflicting interests when they submit their research work. **A conflicting interest does not necessarily mean that the results of a study are void.**

Hepworth SJ, Schoemaker MJ, Muir KR, Swerdlow AJ, van Tongeren MJA, McKinney PA. Mobile phone use and risk of glioma in adults: case-control study. British Medical Journal 2006, 332, 883-7.

Conclusion: The use of a mobile phone is not associated with an increased risk of glioma.

Conflicting interest: The study was partly funded by mobile phone manufacturers.

THE CLINICAL QUESTION

Scenario 2

Dr Green, a General Practitioner, smiled as he read the final draft of his research paper. His survey of 50 patients with fungal nail infections demonstrated that more than half of them had used a public swimming pool in the month before infection. He posted a copy of the paper to his Public Health Consultant, proposing he submit the article to the Journal of Public Health.

A common misconception is that the study design is the most important determinant of the merits of a clinical paper. As soon as the words 'randomised controlled trial' appear, many doctors assume that the study is of great value and the results can be applied to their own medical practice. If this approach was true, then there would be no need for any other type of study.

The critical appraisal of a paper must begin by looking at the clinical question that is at the heart of the paper. **The clinical question determines which study designs can be used to answer that question.**

- One clinical question can be answered by a number of study designs.
- No single study design can answer all clinical questions.

The clinical question

There are five broad categories for clinical questions, as shown in **Table 2**.

CLINICAL QUESTION	CLINICAL RELEVANCE AND POSSIBLE STUDY DESIGNS
Diagnosis	How valid and reliable is a diagnostic test? What does the test tell the doctor? Example: case–control study
Aetiology / causation	What caused the disorder and how is this related to the development of the illness? Example: randomised controlled trial, case–control study, cohort study
Therapy	Which treatments do more good than harm compared with an alternative treatment? Example: randomised controlled trial, systematic review, meta-analysis
Prognosis	What is the likely course of a patient's illness? What is the balance of the risks and benefits of treatments? Example: cohort study, longitudinal survey
Cost effectiveness	Which intervention is worth prescribing? Is newer treatment X worth prescribing compared with older treatment Y? Example: economic analysis

Table 2   The different types of clinical question

Usually, broad questions such as 'how do I treat diabetes mellitus?' and 'what causes bowel cancer?' are easy to understand. These questions are looking for general information.

More specific questions focused on individuals can be more difficult to understand; for example, 'how do I treat hypothyroidism in patients with recurrent depressive disorders and who are receiving lithium therapy?' The acronym 'PICO', explained in **Table 3**, can help you make sense of the question. The other benefit of PICO is that it phrases questions in a way that will direct the search to relevant and precise answers.

P	Patient or Problem	Describe your patient and their problem
I	Intervention	Describe the main intervention, exposure, test or prognostic factor under consideration
C	Comparison	In the case of treatment, describe a comparative intervention. A comparison is not always needed
O	Outcomes	Describe what you hope to achieve, measure or affect

Table 3 Introducing PICO

An example of PICO is shown in **Table 4**.

P	Patient or Problem	In a middle-aged male with schizophrenia …
I	Intervention	… what is the likelihood of olanzapine …
C	Comparison	… compared with haloperidol …
O	Outcomes	… producing fewer extrapyramidal side-effects but similar or better reduction in symptoms?

Table 4 An example of PICO

Scenario 2 revisited

Dr Green's colleague was less enthusiastic about the findings. He wrote, "Interesting though the results are, your chosen study design shows merely an association between swimming pools and fungal nail infections. I think you wanted to know whether a causative relationship exists. I'm afraid a cross-sectional survey cannot answer that question. Before you panic the Great British public, may I suggest you go back to the drawing board and, based on your question, choose a more appropriate study design?"

STUDY DESIGN – OVERVIEW

The type of clinical question determines the types of study that will be appropriate.

Study designs fall into three main categories:

1. **Observational studies (descriptive):** the researcher reports what has been observed in a sample.

2. **Observational studies (analytical):** the researcher reports the similarities and differences observed between two or more samples.

3. **Experimental studies:** the researcher intervenes in some way with the experimental group and reports any differences in the outcome between this experimental group and a control group in which no intervention or a different intervention was offered.

In the next four chapters, examples of study designs that fit into these categories will be given. The advantages and disadvantages of different designs may include references to terms that we have not yet covered. (**Figure 5** on page 23 is a flowchart which can be used to decide study type.)

OBSERVATIONAL STUDIES (DESCRIPTIVE)

In descriptive observational studies, the researcher describes what has been observed in a sample. Nothing is done to the individuals in the sample. These studies are useful for generating hypotheses that can be tested using other study designs.

Survey

A group of people are questioned. Such surveys can identify patterns and help to plan service provision. Surveys cannot distinguish between cause and effect.

Escher M, Perneger TV, Chevrolet JC. National questionnaire survey on what influences doctors' decisions about admission to intensive care. British Medical Journal 2004, 329, 425.

Conclusion: Doctors' decisions to admit patients to intensive care units are influenced by the wishes of patients, patients' personalities and the availability of beds.

Case report

A single patient with the disease is studied. Case reports are easy to write, but they tend to be anecdotal and cannot usually be repeated. They are also prone to chance association and observer bias. Their value lies in the fact that they can be used to generate a hypothesis.

Kassim Z, Sellars M, Greenough A. Underwater birth and neonatal respiratory distress. British Medical Journal 2005, 330, 1071–2.

Summary: A case report highlighting the possibility and adverse effects of aspiration of water by newborns in birthing pools.

Case series

A group of patients are studied. Case series are useful for rare diseases.

Coker WJ, Bhatt BM, Blatchley NF, Graham JT. Clinical findings for the first 1000 Gulf war veterans in the Ministry of Defence's medical assessment programme. British Medical Journal 1999, 318, 290–4.

Conclusion: No single cause has been found to explain the wide variety of symptoms displayed by many Gulf war veterans.

Ecological study

A population or community is studied for associations between the occurrence of disease and exposure to known or suspected causes. Ecological studies can use pre-recorded data. They give information at a population rather than an individual level.

Boydell J, van Os J, McKenzie K, Allardyce J, Goel R, McCreadie RG, et al. Incidence of schizophrenia in ethnic minorities in London: ecological study into interactions with environment. British Medical Journal 2001, 323, 1336.

Conclusion: The incidence of schizophrenia in non-white ethnic minorities in London is greater when they comprise a smaller proportion of the local population.

Qualitative study

Opinions are elicited from a group of people, with the emphasis on the subjective meaning and experience. Such studies can be used to study complex issues. The inquiry can be via interviews, focus groups and participant observation. However, it can be difficult to get information, record it and analyse the subjective data.

Townsend A, Hunt K, Wyke S. Managing multiple morbidity in mid-life: a qualitative study of attitudes to drug use. British Medical Journal 2003, 327, 837.

Conclusion: Involving patients in decisions about their care and a better understanding of patients' experiences of medication regimens will enable doctors to improve rates of compliance.

OBSERVATIONAL STUDIES (ANALYTICAL)

In analytical observational studies, the researcher reports the similarities and differences observed between two or more samples.

Case–control study

Patients who have the outcome variable are compared with individuals who don't have the outcome variable, to find out what risk factors both groups have been exposed to in the past (**Figure 1**). Case–control studies are also known as case comparison or retrospective case–control studies. They are usually quick and cheap to do, as few participants are required. They are particularly valuable in the study of rare diseases or those with a long duration between exposure and outcome or several exposures. They are a good choice for answering clinical questions on diagnosis and aetiology.

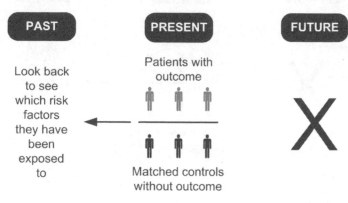

Figure 1: Case–control study design

The main problem with case–control studies is the need to rely on recall and records to determine which risk factors the participants have been exposed to. They are also not good for studying rare exposures, as too many patients with the outcome would be required. The temporal relationship between exposure and outcome may be difficult to establish.

Pierfitte C, Macouillard G, Thicoïpe M, Chaslerie A, Pehourcq F, Aïssou M, et al. Benzodiazepines and hip fractures in elderly people: case–control study. British Medical Journal 2006, 332, 696–700.

Conclusion: Except for lorazepam, the presence of benzodiazepines in plasma was not associated with an increased risk of hip fracture.

Cohort study

Cohort studies are also known as prospective or follow-up studies. A group of people are followed up to see how the development of an outcome differs between groups with and without exposure to a risk factor (**Figure 2**). Such studies are good for resolving questions about aetiology, harm and prognosis. They are suitable for studying rare exposures. They can assess temporal relationships and multiple outcomes. They can also give a direct estimation of disease incidence rates.

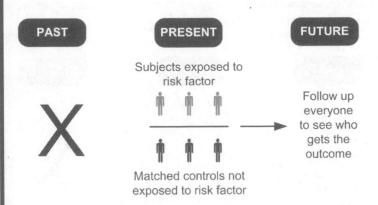

Figure 2: Cohort study design

Cohort studies are unsuitable for studying rare outcomes, as the number of participants required to detect the rare outcome would be large. It may also take a long time from exposure to the development of the outcome. These studies are therefore expensive to set up and maintain. Selection bias becomes a problem if people drop out of the study. Confounding factors can also be a problem. Blinding is difficult and there is no randomisation.

Nielsen NR, Zhang ZF, Kristensen TS, Netterstrøm B, Schnohr P, Grønbæk M. Self reported stress and risk of breast cancer: prospective cohort study. British Medical Journal 2005, 331, 548.

Conclusion: Stress impairs oestrogen synthesis, reducing the risk of breast cancer. However, stress may have other health consequences.

Cross-sectional survey

People who have been exposed to risk factors and the outcome are compared. Such surveys are cheap, simple and are ethically safe. They are useful for establishing prevalence. They establish association, not causality. Recall bias is a problem. The groups may be unequal and confounders may be unequally distributed. Large numbers of subjects are usually required.

Johansen D, Friis K, Skovenborg E, Grønbæk M. Food buying habits of people who buy wine or beer: cross sectional study. British Medical Journal 2006, 332, 519–22.

Conclusions: Wine buyers made more purchases of healthy food items than people who bought beer.

EXPERIMENTAL STUDIES

In experimental studies, the researcher intervenes in some way with the experimental group and reports any differences in the outcome between this experimental group and a control group in whom no intervention or a different intervention was offered.

Open trial
All the people in the study are given the same treatment. In the absence of a control group, these studies are cheap and easy to perform.

Controlled trial
People in the study are given one of two treatments. The absence of randomisation introduces biases in the results.

Pragmatic trial
All the people in a clinical location, such as an outpatient department, are randomly assigned to groups to receive a particular treatment protocol. Allowances for minor differences in the actual treatment may be made. These trials are more reflective of everyday practice and they measure effectiveness. However, they are difficult to control, difficult to make blind, and there is difficulty with excessive drop-outs. To ensure that the results of the trial can be generalised to a wider population, the patients selected should be representative of the patients who will receive the treatment.

Crossover trial
All the people receive one treatment, then switch to the other treatment halfway through the study (**Figure 3**). This can be useful in the study of the treatment of rare diseases. The people in the study are their own controls. There are difficulties with order effects, historical controls and carry-over effects.

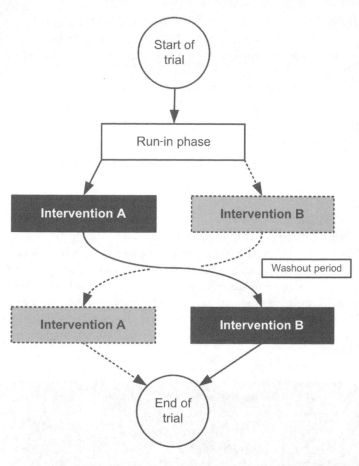

Figure 3: Crossover trial design

Allan L, Hays H, Jensen NH, Polain de Waroux BL, Bolt M, Donald R, et al. Randomised crossover trial of transdermal fentanyl and sustained release oral morphine for treating chronic non-cancer pain. British Medical Journal 2001, 322, 1154.

 Conclusion: Patients with chronic non-cancer pain previously treated with opioids preferred transdermal fentanyl to sustained-release oral morphine.

N of 1 trial

Similar to a crossover design, in a 'N of 1' trial a single person is studied and receives repeated courses of the active drug and placebo in a random order. The patient reports on their progress regularly. This can establish effectiveness in a particular patient, as it can reveal whether clinical improvement occurs only at the time of being in receipt of the active drug.

Cluster trial

In these trials, groups or clusters of people are randomly assigned to study groups instead of individual patients. These trials can be useful to evaluate the delivery of health services.

Randomised controlled trial

People in the study are randomly allocated a treatment, which minimises selection bias and equally distributes confounding factors between the groups. Blinding helps to reduce information bias. Randomised controlled trials are a reliable measure of efficacy and allow for meta-analyses, but they are difficult, time consuming and expensive to set up. There may be ethical problems in giving different treatments to the groups and there is a problem with volunteer bias.

Frost H, Lamb SE, Doll HA, Carver PT, Stewart-Brown S. Randomised controlled trial of physiotherapy compared with advice for low back pain. British Medical Journal 2004, 329, 708.

Conclusion: Routine physiotherapy seemed to be no more effective than one session of assessment and advice from a physiotherapist in the management of low back pain.

The CONSORT statement

Published in Journal of the American Medical Association in August 1996, the CONSORT statement[5] introduced a set of recommendations to improve the quality of randomised controlled trial reports. This checklist is shown in **Table 5**.

5 Moher D, Schulz KF, Altman DG. The CONSORT statement: revised recommendations for improving the quality of reports of parallel-group randomised trials. *Lancet*, 2001, 357, 1191–4.

SECTION OF PAPER	DESCRIPTION
Title & abstract	How participants were allocated to interventions
Introduction	Scientific background and explanation of rationale
Methods	
Participants	Eligibility criteria for participants
Interventions	Details of the interventions for each group
Objectives	Specific objectives and hypotheses
Outcomes	Clearly defined primary and secondary outcome measures
Sample size	How sample size was determined
Randomisation – Sequence generation	Method used to generate the random allocation sequence
Randomisation – Allocation concealment	Method used to implement the random allocation sequence
Randomisation – Implementation	Who generated the allocation sequence, who enrolled participants, and who assigned participants to their groups
Blinding	Whether or not participants, those administering the interventions, and those assessing the outcomes were blinded to group assignment
Statistical methods	Statistical methods used to compare groups for primary outcome(s)
Results	
Participant flow	Flow of participants through each stage
Recruitment	Dates defining the periods of recruitment and follow-up
Baseline data	Baseline demographic and clinical characteristics of each group
Numbers analysed	Number of participants in each group and whether the analysis was by "intention-to-treat"
Outcomes and estimation	For each primary and secondary outcome, a summary of results for each group, and the estimated effect size and its precision

continued

SECTION OF PAPER	DESCRIPTION
Ancillary analyses	Address multiplicity by reporting any other analyses performed
Adverse events	All important adverse events or side-effects in each intervention group
Discussion	
Interpretation	Interpretation of the results
Generalisability	Generalisability (external validity) of the trial findings
Overall evidence	General interpretation of the results in the context of current evidence

Table 5 The CONSORT checklist

OTHER TYPES OF STUDY

Audit

Aspects of service provision are assessed against a gold standard, which can be a national guideline, a local protocol, or generally accepted best practice. Sometimes it is necessary to devise a gold standard, in the absence of a published one.

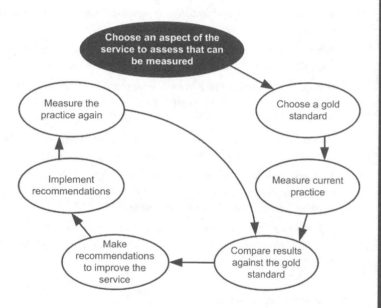

Figure 4: The audit cycle

Data on the service are collected and compared with the gold standard. A change is then implemented in the running of the service and the audit cycle is completed by another collection of data.

Audits give information of the effectiveness of services. However, they are resource-hungry and take clinicians away from clinical work.

Economic analysis

This type of study assesses the cost and/or utilities of intervention. Such analyses help to prioritise services, but it is difficult to remain objective, because assumptions have to be made.

Systematic review and meta-analysis

A systematic review attempts to access and review systematically all of the pertinent articles in the field. A meta-analysis combines the results of several studies and produces a quantitative assessment. Systematic reviews and meta-analyses are discussed in detail on page 96.

Self-assessment exercise 1

What types of studies are suggested by the following statements?

1. Patients with ankle injuries who are seeing a physiotherapist are questioned about the type of trainers they wear in order to investigate the relationship between running shoes and susceptibility to ankle injuries.

2. A group of builders exposed to asbestos on a demolition site are seen regularly, to detect any adverse consequences.

3. A consultant physician investigates how many patients newly referred to the outpatient clinic are seen within 16 weeks of the date of referral.

4. Patients with chronic lower back pain are randomly given one of two treatments and assessed regularly.

5. Residents in a leafy suburb are questioned about their opinions on whether planning permission should be given for a new psychiatric medium-secure unit in the neighbourhood.

6. The Primary Care Trust investigates whether to allocate funds originally set aside for an obesity clinic towards a new treatment for bowel cancer instead.

Self-assessment exercise 2

1. You have developed a blood test for detecting meningitis. How will you set up a study to see if your test is any good?

2. You have developed a new treatment for patients with anorexia nervosa. How will you set up a study to see if your new treatment is any good?

3. You suspect that smoking cannabis leads to the onset of schizophrenia. How will you set up a study to see if this is true?

4. You think that outpatients who are diagnosed with a frozen shoulder will never return to work. How will you set up a study to see if your suspicions are right?

Self-assessment exercise 3

1. What are the advantages and disadvantages of a crossover design compared with a traditional randomised controlled trial?

2. How do cohort studies differ from case–control studies? Which is preferred for investigating the effect of rare exposures? Which is preferred for investigating the cause of rare outcomes?

3. What restriction is imposed on the choice of topics that you as a clinician can audit?

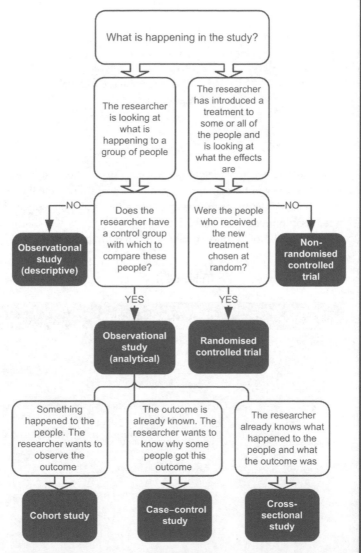

Figure 5: Distinguishing different study designs

THE HIERARCHY OF EVIDENCE

There is a well established hierarchy of research methodologies. The hierarchy is based on the premise that the study designs differ in their ability to predict what will happen to patients in real life. The studies at the top of the hierarchy carry more weight than studies lower down, because their evidence is of a higher grade.

Systematic review
Meta-analysis
Randomised controlled trial
Non-randomised control trial
Cohort studies
Cross-sectional studies
Case series
Case report

Studies that carry more weight are not necessarily the best in every situation, and are unlikely to be appropriate for all situations. For example, a case report can be of great importance, even though in terms of the hierarchy of studies, a case report normally carries the least weight. Also note that the hierarchy is for guidance only; not all studies using the same design are of equal quality.

The NHS Centre for Reviews and Dissemination (CRD) has published its view of the hierarchy of evidence (**Table 6**)[6].

STUDY DESIGN HIERARCHY	
Level	Description
1	Experimental studies (eg, randomised controlled trial with concealed allocation)
2	Quasi-experimental studies (eg, experimental study without randomisation)
3	Controlled observational studies 3a. Cohort studies 3b. Case–control studies
4	Observational studies without control groups
5	Expert opinion based on pathophysiology, bench research or consensus

Table 6   CRD guidelines on the hierarchy of evidence

The National Institute for Clinical Excellence (NICE) also publishes guidance, which is evidence based[7]. It grades its recommendations in a similar way (**Table 7**).

STUDY DESIGN HIERARCHY	
Level	Description
A	Based on level I evidence (meta-analysis of randomised controlled trials or at least one randomised controlled trial)
B	Based on level II or level III evidence (well-conducted clinical studies, but no randomised controlled trials) or extrapolated from level I evidence
C	Based on level IV evidence (expert committee reports or opinions and/or clinical experience of respected authorities)
GPP	Recommended good practice based on clinical experience of the Guideline Development Group
N	Evidence from NICE technology appraisal guidance

Table 7 Grading of recommendations from NICE

6 University of York, NHS Centre for Reviews and Dissemination. *Undertaking systematic reviews of research on effectiveness: CRD Guidelines for those carrying out or commissioning reviews.* CRD Report Number 4 (2nd Edition) March 2001.
7 NICE website: http://www.nice.org.uk/

RESEARCH PATHWAY

Bringing a drug to the market may take several years and cost hundreds of millions of pounds (**Figure 6**). The developmental process usually begins with the identification of a biological target that is linked with the aetiology of a disease. Compounds are formulated to act on this target. The chosen compound is then transformed and packaged in such a way that it can be administered to patients to give the maximum benefit and the minimum of side-effects. This transformation process involves a series of trials on animals and humans that are subject to the rigorous controls required by the regulatory authorities and local ethics committees.

Clinical trial authorisations are needed for all new products in development. Applications for such authorisations in the United Kingdom are assessed by the medical, pharmaceutical and scientific staff at the Medicines and Healthcare products Regulatory Agency (MHRA), an agency of the Department of Health.

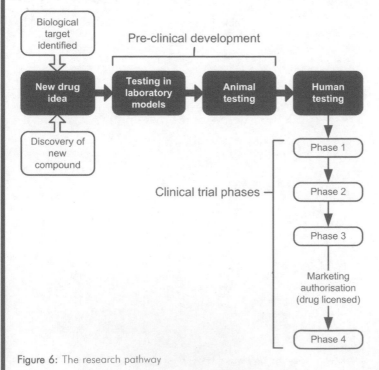

Figure 6: The research pathway

Clinical trial phases

Clinical trials of experimental drugs consist of four phases.

Phase 1 clinical trials

These are the earliest trials in the life of a new drug or treatment. The researchers test a new drug or treatment in a small group of **healthy** people for the first time, to assess its safety, establish a dosage range and identify any side-effects. These trials aim to help in the evaluation and understanding of the behaviour of the molecule or compound. The healthy volunteers are normally recompensed for the time they are giving up, but are not given financial incentives to take part in research.

Phase 2 clinical trials

About 7 out of every 10 new treatments tested at Phase 1 in healthy volunteers proceed to Phase 2 trials and are tested on people with the relevant **illness**. At this stage, the study drug or treatment is given to a larger group of people, to assess its effectiveness and safety profile.

Phase 3 clinical trials

At this stage, the study drug or treatment is given to large groups of people in **clinical settings** to make further assessments of its effectiveness, dose range and duration of treatment, and to monitor side-effects. These trials compare the new treatment with the best currently available treatment (the standard treatment).

Providing satisfactory results are gained from Phase 3 studies, a drug will get a **marketing authorisation**, which sets out its agreed terms and conditions of use, such as indications and dosage. Even drugs with a high risk-to-benefit ratio may be approved if the drug enhances the quality of life of, for example, patients with terminal illnesses.

Phase 4 clinical trials

Phase 4 trials, also known as post-marketing surveillance studies, are carried out after a drug has been shown to work, granted a license and marketed. Information is collected about the benefits and side-effects of the drug in different populations. Data on long-term usage are also collected. These studies involve monitoring the safety of medicines under their usual conditions of use, and can also be carried out to identify any new safety concerns (**hypothesis generating**) and to confirm or refute these concerns (**hypothesis testing**).

SECTION B
METHODOLOGY

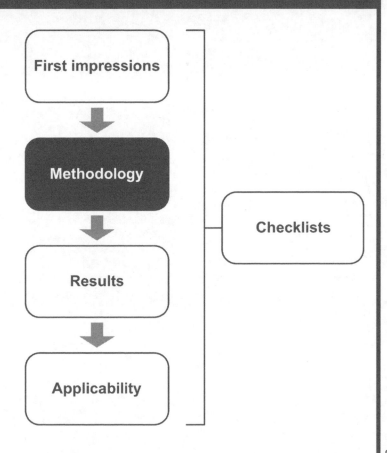

PRIMARY HYPOTHESIS

The type of clinical question determines the types of study that will be appropriate. In the methodology, the researcher must specify how the study will answer the clinical question. This will usually involve stating a hypothesis and then explaining how this hypothesis will be proven or not proven. The hypothesis is usually the same as or closely related to the clinical question.

A study should, ideally, be designed and powered to answer one well-defined hypothesis.

If there is a secondary hypothesis, its analysis needs to be described in the same way as that for the primary hypothesis. The protocol should include details of how the secondary outcomes will be analysed. Ideally, further exploratory analyses should be identified before the completion of the study, and there should be a clear rationale for the reason and value of such analyses.

Finally, not all studies are designed to test a hypothesis. Some studies, such as case reports or qualitative studies, can be used to generate hypotheses.

Self-assessment exercise 4
A study fails to meet its primary hypothesis but it is statistically significant for its secondary and tertiary hypotheses. What conclusions will you draw?

POPULATIONS AND SAMPLES

Researchers identify the target population they are interested in. It may not be feasible to include everyone in the population in the trial. A sample is therefore taken from this population. Results from this sample are then generalised to the target population (**Figure 7**).

There are several sampling techniques that are used to obtain a sample from a population. People could be chosen at random, on the basis of a characteristic, or simply invited because they are known to the researchers.

It is important that the sample is representative of the population it came from. Knowing the **baseline characteristics** of the sample population is important, as it allows doctors to see how closely the members match their own patients. Such characteristics can include demographic characteristics, such as age and sex, as well as more fluid variables, such as smoking status.

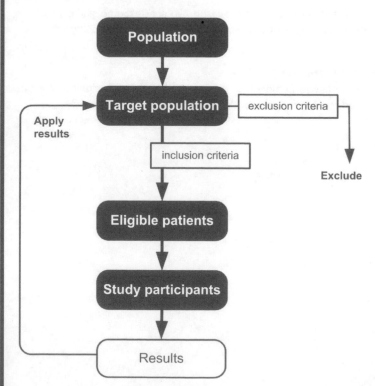

Figure 7: Describing people at different stages of a study

Scenario 3

Dr Pahal, Consultant Orthopaedic Surgeon, was interested in how many patients would use a hospital website to access information about postoperative care. He placed an advertisement in The Times newspaper and recruited 90 people for his survey. He concluded that 85% of patients would definitely visit a hospital website for more information about the management of bone injuries. He put forward a proposal to the Hospital Board for funding the development of such a website.

Scenario 4

Consultant Psychiatrist, Dr Thomas, had a long-standing interest in the treatment of anxiety disorders. His Clinical Director wanted him to set up a specialist clinic for patients with anxiety disorders, but needed to justify the expense involved to the Hospital Board. Dr Thomas sent a postal questionnaire to 500 patients of the psychiatry unit, asking them if they had ever been told they had a neurotic disorder. If the answer was yes, he asked them to describe the treatments offered and whether they would support the development of a specialist clinic.

Errors in studies may lead to results that are misleading and conclusions that are wrong. Interventions and treatments may appear more promising or less beneficial than they actually are. Errors in studies can happen either by chance or through mistakes in the way the study was done.

Bias is used to describe an error (at any stage of the study) that was not due to chance, and therefore it cannot be measured or controlled for statistically. Researchers need to rely on good research techniques to reduce bias as much as possible.

There are numerous types of bias. The main types of bias can be listed either at the stage of the study at which they arise or in the broad categories of reporting, selection, performance, observation and attrition bias (**Table 8**).

STAGE OF STUDY	CATEGORIES OF BIAS	EXAMPLES OF BIAS	EXAMPLES OF AVOIDING BIAS
Literature review	Reporting	Literature search bias Foreign language exclusion bias	Comprehensive search strategy Translation
Recruitment of a sample population	Selection	Sampling bias (researcher): - Berkson bias - diagnostic purity bias - Neyman bias - membership bias - historical control bias Response bias (subjects)	Randomisation Concealed allocation
Running the trial	Performance	Instrument bias Questionnaire bias	Blinding
Collecting data	Observation	Interviewer bias Recall bias Response bias Hawthorne effect	Blinding outcome assessment
Analysing the results	Attrition	Attrition (exclusion) bias	Intention-to-treat analysis

Table 8   The different types of bias

Selection bias

This occurs through the identification and/or recruitment of an unrepresentative sample population. The sample population differs in some significant way from the population that generated the sample population, such that any results and conclusions drawn from the sample population cannot be generalised to the population as a whole. This is a potential problem for all studies.

Selection bias can be further divided into sampling bias, which is introduced by the researchers, or response bias, which is introduced by the study population.

Examples of **sampling bias** include:

> **Berkson (admission) bias:** this arises when the sample population is taken from a hospital setting, but the hospital cases do not reflect the rate or severity of the condition in the population. The relationship between exposure and disease is unrepresentative of the real situation.
>
> **Diagnostic purity bias:** This arises when co-morbidity is excluded in the sample population, such that the sample population does not reflect the true complexity of cases in the population.
>
> **Neyman (incidence / prevalence) bias:** This occurs when the prevalence of a condition does not reflect its incidence. Usually this is due to a time gap between exposure and the actual selection of the study population, such that some individuals with the exposure are not available for selection.
>
> **Membership bias:** This arises when membership of a group is used to identify study individuals. The members of such a group may not be representative of the population.
>
> **Historical control bias:** This arises when subjects and controls are chosen across time, such that secular changes in definitions, exposures, diseases and treatments may mean that such subjects and controls cannot be compared with one another.

Response bias occurs when individuals volunteer for studies but they differ in some way from the population. The most common reason for such a difference is that the volunteers are more motivated to improve their health and therefore participate more readily and adhere to the trial conditions better. Confusingly, the term 'response bias' can also be used to describe an observation bias (see below).

Performance bias

This occurs when individuals in the sample population behave in a certain way because of knowledge of the group they have been allocated to. If they prefer a particular intervention, this may bias an outcome. If subjects are in a group they like and the treatment is effective, they perform better. If the subjects are in a group they dislike and the treatment is ineffective, then it really is ineffective.

Observation bias

Observation bias occurs as a result of failure to measure or classify the exposure or disease correctly. It can be due to the researchers or the subjects.

Examples of observation bias include:

Interviewer (ascertainment) bias: This arises when the researcher is not blinded to the subject's status in the study and this alters the researcher's approach to the subject and the recording of results.

Recall bias: This arises when subjects selectively remember details from the past. This can be particularly important in case–control studies and cross-sectional surveys.

Response bias: This arises in any study in which the subjects are asked questions, if the subjects answer questions in the way they believe the researcher wants them to answer, rather than according to their true beliefs.

Hawthorne effect: This arises when subjects alter their behaviour, usually positively, because they are aware they are being observed in a study.

Attrition bias

Attrition bias arises when the numbers of individuals dropping out of the study differ significantly in the different arms of the study. Those left at the end of the study may not be representative of the study sample that was randomised at the start.

Scenario 3 revisited

Dr Pahal's proposal was rejected by the Hospital Board. In their conclusions, they commented: "A non-representative sample was used to generate the findings. The population that the hospital serves is dissimilar to that which reads The Times newspaper in a number of respects, including, but not limited to, lower literacy levels and less Internet access. Dr Pahal should consider selecting a more representative sample for future proposals, to avoid selection bias."

Scenario 4 revisited

Dr Thomas's survey generated a surprising result, with only 1% of the sample having been diagnosed with a neurotic disorder. His Clinical Director wrote to him, stating that, "Perhaps not many people are familiar with the term 'neurotic'. The use of the word 'anxiety' may produce different results as it will eliminate observation bias. Please repeat the survey."

Self-assessment exercise 5

For each of the following study protocols, decide if selection and/or observation bias may occur.

1. **Study aim:** To plan the provision of stroke services for elderly patients.

   Proposed method: A cross-sectional survey to discover the prevalence of cerebrovascular accidents by phoning 5000 residents across the city.

2. **Study aim:** To elicit the magnitude of drug problems in the teenage population.

   Proposed method: A survey of teenagers in all the schools in the city, asking them about illicit use of drugs.

3. **Study aim:** To investigate the association between smoking and lung cancer.

   Proposed method: A case–control study of inpatients in a respiratory disease ward in a district general hospital.

4. **Study aim:** To establish the effectiveness of pain relief offered to women during childbirth.

   Proposed method: A questionnaire sent to new mothers asking them about their experience of pain during delivery.

CONFOUNDING FACTORS

Scenario 5

Dr Edwards designed a case–control study to investigate the relationship between alcohol consumption and lung cancer. He recruited 700 people, both healthy controls and lung cancer sufferers, into his study. He questioned each person on their alcohol history. To his surprise he found a significant relationship, showing that alcohol consumption increased the risk of lung cancer, such that the finding was unlikely to have happened by chance alone. He submitted his article to the British Medical Journal.

Many studies look at the relationship between an exposures and an outcome, hoping to show whether a causal relationship exists. The findings may, however, be explained by the existence of a third factor, a confounder.

A confounder has a triangular relationship with both the exposure and the outcome, but most importantly, it is not on the causal pathway (**Figure 8**). It makes it appear as if there is a direct relationship between the exposure and the outcome, or it may even mask an association that would otherwise have been present.

A **positive confounder** results in an association between two variables that are not associated.

A **negative confounder** masks an association which is really present.

To be a confounding factor, the variable must be associated with:

1. the exposure but not be the consequence of the exposure, and

2. the outcome, independently of the exposure (ie, not an intermediary).

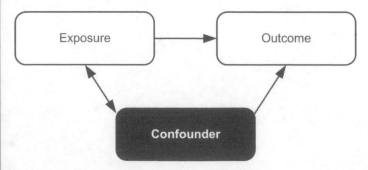

Figure 8: The relationship between the exposure, the outcome and the confounder

THE DOCTOR'S GUIDE TO CRITICAL APPRAISAL

In the example below (**Figure 9**), drinking coffee appears to cause coronary heart disease. Smoking is a confounding factor. It is associated with coffee drinking and it is a risk factor for coronary heart disease, even in people who do not drink coffee.

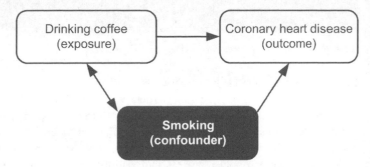

Figure 9: Smoking is a confounding factor

The reverse is not true. Coffee drinking does not confound the relationship between smoking and coronary heart disease, even though it is associated with smoking. Drinking coffee is not a risk factor for coronary heart disease independently of smoking (**Figure 10**).

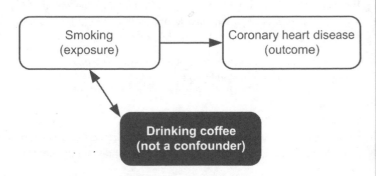

Figure 10: Drinking coffee is not a confounding factor

Confounding factors differ from bias in that confounding is not created by some mistake made by the researchers and therefore cannot be controlled by better research techniques. Confounding arises from a real-life relationship that already exists between the exposures being examined and outcomes under consideration. Importantly, confounding factors must be identified so that measures can be taken to eliminate them, spread them equally between different arms of the study, or neutralise their effects on the results using statistical techniques.

In the study design	In the analysis
Restriction Matching Randomisation	Stratification Multivariate statistics

Table 9   Methods to reduce confounding

There are several methods by which we can reduce confounding at the study design stage or at the analysis stage (**Table 9**). Confounding factors can be measured and controlled for by multiple linear regression, for example. It is important to remember that one of the key strengths of randomised controlled trials is that, because of the randomisation, they are free of baseline confounding factors. Another process that will also ensure that there are no subsequent confounding factors during the trial is complete blinding. Finally, confounders can exert effects only if they differ between study groups.

Restriction

Inclusion and exclusion criteria are introduced so that the confounding factor is **eliminated** altogether in the sample population.

The inclusion and exclusion of patients will influence the generalisability of the results. Over-restriction of the sample population should be avoided, otherwise the sample population will not be representative of the population.

In order to minimise selection bias, the inclusion and exclusion criteria must be clearly stated before the study begins.

Inclusion criteria

These depend on the question being asked, diagnosis and demographics; for example age, setting, illness characteristics, treatment characteristics, etc.

Exclusion criteria

This is a balance between a highly selected group with little generalisability and an unselected heterogeneous group.

Matching

Study participants are chosen to ensure that potential confounding variables are **evenly distributed** in the two groups being compared. This ensures that any confounding factor that has been identified in the experimental group can also be replicated in the control group. Matching must be used with caution as it can, like restriction, limit the sample size and possible analysis strategies.

Randomisation

This method ensures that all the individuals entering into a study have an equal chance of being allocated to any group within the study. As a result of randomisation, confounding factors, known and unknown, have an equal chance of entering either group. Allocation of participants to specific treatment groups in a random fashion ensures that each group is, on average, as alike as possible to the other group(s). Successful randomisation requires that group assignment cannot be predicted in advance.

Randomisation can be divided into:

- **Fixed randomisation:** here, the randomisation methods (eg, simple randomisation, block randomisation, stratified randomisation and randomised consent) are defined, and allocation sequences are set up, before the start of the trial.

- **Adaptive randomisation:** here, the randomised groups are adjusted as the study progresses, to account for imbalances in the numbers in the groups or in response to the outcome data. Minimisation is an example of adaptive randomisation.

Randomisation can be divided into three broad areas that all overlap:

- sequence generation

- concealed allocation

- implementation.

The method of generating the random number sequence can differ according to the study design. The trial statistician usually generates the randomisation sequence. A good study should indicate who generated the sequence, the method used, and how concealment was achieved and monitored. There may also be a table in a methodology section of the paper that compares the major baseline demographic and prognostic characteristics of the two groups.

Some methods of allocation such as alternate allocation to treatment group, or methods based on patient characteristics are not reliably random. These allocation sequences are predictable and not easily concealed, and therefore may reduce the guarantee that allocation has been random, and that no potential participants have been excluded by pre-existing knowledge of the intervention.

Concealed allocation

It is important that randomisation is adhered to at the time of treatment allocation. This is done by concealing the imminent allocation from those responsible for recruiting people into a trial, so that they are unaware of the group to which a participant will be allocated, should that individual agree to be in the study. As a result, you can ensure that the researcher's knowledge of the patient cannot influence the selection procedure. This avoids both conscious and unconscious selection of patients into the study. 'Concealed allocation' is the term used to describe this process.

Concealed allocation can be achieved with central concealment, for example telephone, Internet or pharmacy concealment. This can be used, for example, with multi-centre clinical trials. The clinician checks for eligibility, gains consent, decides on whether to enrol patients, and then calls the randomisation service to obtain the treatment allocation. As a result, central randomisation allows you to have a record of all allocated patients for potential follow-up and holds information on randomisation rates.

Other methods include using sealed envelopes. For example, with single-centre clinical trials, you can have a randomisation list or envelopes, in a location away from the clinic where patients are being assessed. Pharmacy staff may be able to undertake the randomisation. In situations in which remote randomisation may not be feasible, a set of tamper-evident envelopes that look identical may be provided to each site. The envelopes are opaque and well sealed, and the sequence of opening the envelopes is monitored regularly.

Methods of randomisation

Simple randomisation (these methods are simple and commonly used with large samples)

- Flipping a coin (for studies with two groups)
- Rolling a dice (for studies with two or more groups)
- Random number tables and computer-generated random numbers.

Block randomisation

In small trials, simple randomisation may not give well balanced groups. Block randomisation is used to ensure that equal numbers of patients are in each arm. The 'blocks' comprise equal numbers of individuals who will go into the experimental and control groups. The order of this allocation into experimental and control groups within the block is randomly permuted. Some clinical papers refer to this method as 'permuted block randomisation'. A random number sequence is used to choose a particular block for each set of individuals.

Stratification

If a potential confounding factor can be identified in the design stage, the data generated during the study can be separated into strata based on that potential confounding factor. This enables the researcher to keep the characteristics of the participants as similar as possible across the study groups (eg, age, weight or functional status). Once these strata are identified, separate block randomisation schemes are created for each factor, to ensure that the groups are balanced within each stratum.

Stratification can be achieved by a statistical technique called the Mantel–Haenszel method, which gives adjusted relative risks as a summary measure of the overall risk, or the Mantel–Haenszel estimate of odds ratio, which gives a weighted average of the strata specific odds ratios, the weights being dependent upon the numbers of observations in each stratum.

Multivariate statistics and confounding factors

This statistical method is used to take confounding factors into account. It analyses the data by using a mathematical model that takes the outcome under consideration as the dependent variable and includes the causal factor and any confounding factors in the equation. These factors are referred to as 'covariables'. The equation allows you to check how much the confounding factors / covariables contribute to the overall effect. When the dependent variables are continuous in nature, multiple linear regression is used. If the variables are binary, logistic regression is used.

Scenario 5 revisited

Dr Edwards received a letter from the editor of the British Medical Journal. The editor wrote, "Although a most interesting conclusion, the results of the study are less impressive when confounding variables are considered. Unfortunately, smoking as a confounder has been overlooked. I'm afraid that we cannot consider publishing your study results. I wish you better luck in the future."

Self-assessment exercise 6

1. In the following lists of three variables, state which factor, if not identified, would act as a confounding factor in the relationship between the other two variables:

   a. Cigarette lighter; smoking cigarettes; lung cancer.
   b. Skin cancer; fair skin; blue eyes.
   c. Smoking; the oral contraceptive pill; myocardial infarction.
   d. Life events; poverty; depression.

2. You are developing a study protocol looking at the benefits of the antipsychotic drug, risperidone, in the treatment of schizoaffective disorder in hospital inpatients. Which inclusion and exclusion criteria would you apply?

BLINDING

Scenario 6

Dr Singh, a rheumatologist, finished writing his first case report. He had seen a patient with arthritis. The patient had visited his general practitioner and had, by the press of a wrong key on the computer, been mistakenly dispensed co-careldopa, a treatment for Parkinson's disease, instead of co-codamol, a pain killer. The patient had unwittingly taken the wrong treatment for a month and, far from experiencing no effect, the patient had dramatically improved pain symptoms. Dr Singh submitted his report to The Lancet, stating that for the first time the pain-killing properties of anti-Parkinsonism treatment had been demonstrated, and may lead to a new treatment approach.

Scenario 7

Dr Joseph analysed the results of a trial on the usefulness of psychological interventions in patients suffering chronic pain. In one arm of the study, the patients received 20 weekly sessions with a psychologist, exploring their perceptions of pain. In the control arm, the patients were invited to chat to a nurse about their daily routine. The psychologists dramatically reduced pain scores compared with the 'placebo' intervention. Dr Joseph wrote to his Hospital Board, suggesting that sessions with psychologists were a cost-effective intervention for his patients and may reduce the need for pain clinic appointments.

Placebo response

A placebo is a dummy intervention that does not have any therapeutic activity for the condition being treated. Placebos are used in trials to learn if any differences observed are attributable to the intervention under investigation or to the power of suggestion. Usually, one arm of the study will receive the intervention, while the other arm will receive a placebo.

The power of suggestion may cause symptoms to improve. For example, by giving a patient a pill and telling them it is a pain-killer, the pain reported by the patient may be reduced. Similarly, several pills are seen to be more effective than single pills, larger pills are better than smaller pills, and capsules are seen as stronger than tablets. The response rates to placebo interventions can be very high. In any trial, comparison with placebo treatment is essential.

Blinding

The behaviour of researchers and study participants can be influenced by what they know or believe. If participants in a trial are aware they are receiving a placebo or active intervention, the answers they give may be influenced by this knowledge. Similarly, the researchers may also be influenced by any awareness of which individuals are receiving the different interventions. The behaviour of study participants and researchers may lead to bias, as the subjective answers and assessments may not actually mirror the truth. Blinding is used to overcome this.

- **Single blinding:** Either the researcher or the subject is blind to the allocation.

- **Double blinding:** The subject and the researcher are unaware of the treatment being administered. Differences in taste, smell or mode of delivery should be identical for each treatment group.

- **Triple blinding:** Knowledge of the treatment is concealed from the patients, investigators and the analyst processing the results.

If the interventions are very different, a **double-dummy** technique may be used, in which all the subjects appear to receive both interventions, although one is a placebo, in order to maintain blinding.

The blinding procedure should be clearly stated in the methodology section of the study. As a result of blinding, the groups in the trial should be treated equally.

Treatment is termed 'blind' when the patient and/or investigator do not know what trial treatments are being administered.

Blind assessment is assessment of the outcome measures during and at the end of the study, without any knowledge of what the treatment groups are.

Scenario 6 revisited

The editor of The Lancet wrote back to Dr Singh. He thanked Dr Singh for submitting his case report but noted that, "The placebo effect of co-careldopa needs to be explored and will probably explain the beneficial effects seen. To really demonstrate the efficacy of co-careldopa with pain symptoms, I would suggest a placebo-controlled double-blind strategy is more appropriate. I'll be happy to publish these results if they can be replicated in a better study."

Scenario 7 revisited

The Medical Director of the hospital wrote back to Dr Joseph, stating, "It is hardly surprising that the psychotherapy patients got better. They were aware they were getting the new intervention. While I accept that talking therapies are hard to blind, we mustn't rush into making costly decisions based on such trials."

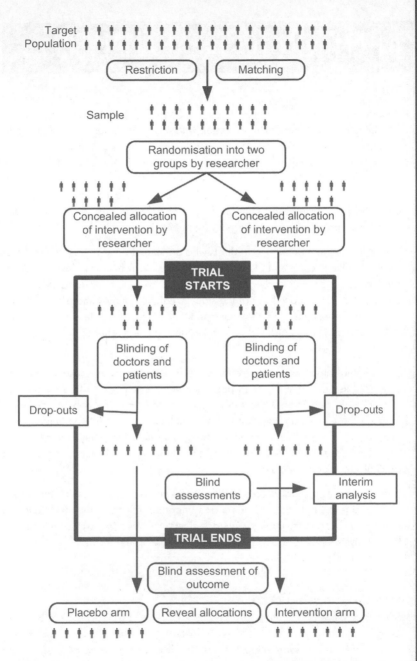

Figure 11: The study pathway

INTENTION-TO-TREAT ANALYSIS

Scenario 8

Dr Franks returned from his lunch break with renewed vigour. He had just read the conclusion of a trial on the treatment of ear infections in children using a new antibiotic, zapitillin, compared with his usual choice, amoxicillin. In the zapitillin arm, 240 out of 300 children who completed the study improved (80%). In the amoxicillin arm, 300 out of 400 children who completed the study improved (71%). He sent a copy of the paper to his colleague, proposing that zapitillin be first choice in the hospital formulary.

In most studies some of the individuals who are eligible and participate in a trial may not make it to the end of the trial. There are many reasons why such '**drop-outs**' occur, including early deaths, loss to follow-up (individuals cannot be contacted or have moved out of the study area), voluntary withdrawal from the trial, non-compliance with the trial conditions, and ineligible patients. Some individuals may also not be able to take the treatments offered to them in the trial.

Determining the sample of patients to be analysed is a key step in reporting clinical trials. Ideally, a research paper should account for all its subjects who were eligible and started the trial, explaining the reasons behind some not finishing the trial. In an **intention-to-treat analysis**, all the study participants are included in the analyses as part of the groups to which they are allocated, regardless of whether they completed the study or not. It keeps them in the original groups for the purpose of statistical analysis.

If these patients are not accounted for in the analysis of the results, the results and conclusions may be misleading and important effects of the intervention in terms of, for example, intolerable side-effects, can be lost. Exclusion from the final analysis leads to a bias in the interpretation of the results. This is referred to as attrition bias (also known as exclusion bias).

Handling missing data

Steps to achieve an intention-to-treat analysis should be considered in both the design and conduct of a trial. Any eligibility errors can be avoided by careful inspection before random allocation. Efforts should be made to ensure minimal drop-outs from treatment and losses to follow-up. In some studies, an active run-in phase is introduced at the start of the study and this can help identify patients who are likely to drop out.

During the trial, continuing clinical support should be available to all participants.

If drop-outs occur in a study, the researcher has to decide how to include these individuals in an intention-to-treat analysis. With luck, some data will have been collected up to the point at which these subjects left the trial. Ideally, data on the primary endpoints are collected after drop out.

- In **last observation carried forward**, the last recorded results of individuals who drop out are carried forward to the end of the trial and incorporated into the final analysis of the results.

- In **sensitivity analysis**, assumptions are made when the missing values are put in. Sensitivity analyses can also be carried out to include different scenarios of assumptions, such as the worst-case and best-case scenarios. Worst-case scenario sensitivity analysis is performed by assigning the worst outcomes to the missing patients in the group who show the best results. These results are then compared with the initial analysis, which excludes the missing data.

- In studies that have many drop-outs, the **drop-out event** itself should be considered as an important endpoint.

It is important to establish whether the reasons drop-outs are no longer taking part are in some way attributable to the intervention. The chance of there being drop-outs should be minimised early on when the study is being planned and during trial monitoring.

Utilisation of 'last observation carried forward' can lead to underestimation or overestimation of treatment effects.

Figure 12 shows the result of treating a depressed patient with an antidepressant. Over the trial, the patient's depressive symptoms improve gradually, such that, at the end of the trial, they were less depressed than at the start.

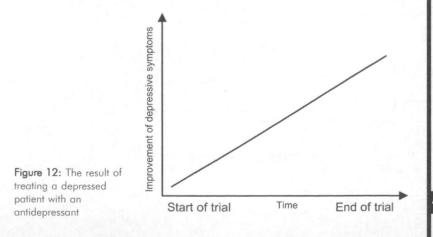

Figure 12: The result of treating a depressed patient with an antidepressant

If a different individual dropped out of the study at an early stage and the last observation was carried forward, the results may underestimate the true effect of the antidepressant, which would have been apparent had the individual completed the trial (**Figure** 13).

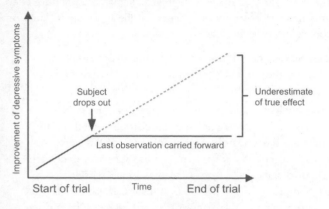

Figure 13: Underestimation of the treatment effect

Overestimation of a treatment effect may occur with last observation carried forward in conditions that normally deteriorate with time.

Figure 14 shows the results of the Mini-Mental State Examination score of a dementing individual being treated with an anti-dementia drug. Over the trial, their dementia will progress, but at a slower rate with treatment.

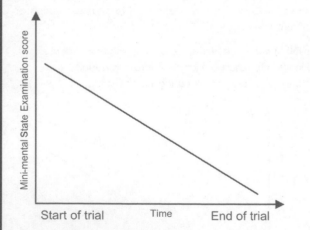
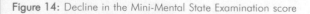

Figure 14: Decline in the Mini-Mental State Examination score

If a different individual drops out of the trial at an early stage, the effects of the anti-dementia drug in delaying the progression of dementia may be over-stated (**Figure 15**).

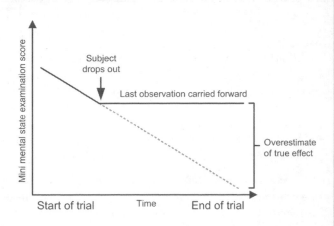

Figure 15: Overestimation of treatment effect

Per-protocol analysis

A per-protocol or on-treatment analysis is an approach used in which data from only those patients who sufficiently complied with the trial protocol are considered in the analysis. The disadvantage of this method is that it can introduce bias related to excluding participants from analysis. Therefore, the intention-to-treat analysis should always be considered as the analysis of choice, and if necessary the study could have a secondary analysis using the per-protocol approach.

Scenario 8 revisited

Dr Franks' colleague read the paper too, but came to a different conclusion. He emailed Dr Franks, "I disagree with the conclusions the researchers have drawn. Five hundred patients were enrolled into each arm of the study. I worked out that the results did not take into account the drop-outs in both arms. Intention-to-treat analysis shows that amoxicillin gave better results, with 300 children out of 500 children improving (60%). In contrast, only 240 children improved with zapitillin (48%). I won't be prescribing zapitillin unless the child has an allergy to amoxicillin, but thanks for drawing my attention to the paper."

RELIABILITY

Scenario 9

Dr Nolan was supervising a class of first-year medical students. All the students were asked to take each others' blood pressure until they were comfortable using a sphygmomanometer. Dr Nolan noticed that, halfway through the session, some of the students looked bemused. He asked one student what the matter was. "It's these sphygmomanometers," said the student, "they never give the same result twice!" After the session, Dr Nolan wrote to the Clinical Tutor, suggesting that an investment be made in better equipment.

Many studies involve the measurement of one or more variables. Good research technique involves commenting on the reliability of these measurements – that is, the consistency of test results on repeat measurements. Repeat measurements can be by the same person, by more than one person, and/or across time. Good reliability ensures consistency of the results and conclusions that are being drawn from the study.

Test–retest reliability: Refers to the level of agreement between the initial test results and the results of repeat measurements made at a later date.

Inter-rater reliability: Refers to the level of agreement between assessments made by two or more raters at the same time. This measure of agreement can be quantified as a correlation coefficient, the Kappa (Cohen's) statistic (κ). Kappa is also known as the chance-corrected proportional agreement statistic.

Measurements can agree purely by chance. The Kappa statistic (κ) indicates the level of the agreement between measurements by different raters and gives an indication as to whether this agreement is more than can be expected by chance. If agreement is no more than expected by chance, then $\kappa = 0$. With perfect agreement, $\kappa = 1$ (**Table 10**). To avoid low Kappa values, measurements by researchers can be improved by simply agreeing criteria and measurement conditions. One disadvantage of this measurement of agreement is that it is sensitive to the prevalence / proportion of individuals in each group.

To calculate Kappa:

$$\kappa = (P_O - P_E) / (1 - P_E)$$

P_O = observed agreement

P_E = agreement expected by chance.

KAPPA	STRENGTH OF AGREEMENT
0	Chance agreement only
<0.2	Poor agreement beyond chance
0.21–0.4	Fair agreement beyond chance
0.41–0.6	Moderate agreement beyond chance
0.61–0.8	Good agreement beyond chance
0.81–1.0	Very good agreement beyond chance
1.0	Perfect agreement

Table 10 Kappa (κ) and the strength of agreement

Kappa is for use with tests measuring categorical variables. For nominal-ordered data, Kappa is preferably weighted (κw) to allow for any near misses.

Cronbach's α: This is used with complicated tests with several parts or for measuring several variables. If Cronbach's $\alpha \geq 0.5$ there is moderate agreement and ≥ 0.8 is excellent agreement.

Intraclass correlation coefficient: This is for use with tests measuring quantitative variables. It describes the extent to which two continuous measures taken by different people, or two measurements taken by the same person on different occasions, are related.

Other types of reliability include:

Intra-rater reliability: This looks at the level of agreement between assessments by one rater of the same material at two or more different times.

Alternative-form reliability: This describes reliability of similar forms of the test, looking at the same material either at the same time or immediately consecutively. For example, the temperature reading from a mercury thermometer may be compared with that from a digital thermometer.

Split-half reliability: This describes the reliability of a test that is divided in two, with each half being used to assess the same material under similar circumstances.

Scenario 9 revisited

The Clinical Tutor wrote back to Dr Nolan, thanking him for his feedback. He went on, "The issue of reliability is indeed an important one in blood pressure measurements. I don't think simply having a new set of sphygmomanometers will make much of a difference, because the reliability of the measure is never going to be perfect, no matter who uses the sphygmomanometer!"

Scenario 10

Dr Harrison looked at the next research proposal submitted for ethics approval. A junior doctor wished to compare the efficacy of a new thyroxine depot injection against that of thyroxine tablets, in young men with hypothyroidism. He proposed a cohort study assessing the severity of symptoms by the television viewing time of each subject at home, as hypothyroid patients tended to be tired all the time. He hypothesised that thyroxine treatment would improve hypothyroid symptoms, marked by a reduction in the amount of television viewed.

The term '**validity**' refers to the extent to which a test measures what it is supposed to measure. There are many subtypes of validity.

Criterion validity

This is made up of predictive, concurrent, convergent and discriminant validity. It is used to demonstrate the accuracy of a measure or procedure by comparing it with another measure or procedure that has been demonstrated to be valid.

Predictive validity: The extent to which the test is able to predict something it should theoretically be able to predict. For example, a written examination would have predictive validity if it measured performance in high school and successfully predicted employment status in adulthood.

Concurrent validity: The extent to which the test is able to distinguish between groups it should theoretically be able to distinguish between. For example, a questionnaire would have concurrent validity if it successfully distinguished sufferers of chest pain due to angina from sufferers of chest pain due to gastritis.

Convergent validity: The extent to which the test is similar to other tests that it theoretically should be similar to. For example, a digital thermometer would have convergent validity with a mercury-based thermometer if it returned similar results.

Discriminant validity: The extent to which the test is not similar to other tests that it theoretically should not be similar to. For example, a postgraduate assessment of critical appraisal skills of doctors would have discriminant validity if it returned results dissimilar to a multiple-choice question paper testing knowledge of disease.

Other types of validity include:

Face validity: The extent to which the test, on superficial consideration, measures what it is supposed to measure. For example, a test measuring the exercise tolerance of patients and relating it to respiratory disease severity would have face validity.

Content validity: The extent to which the test measures variables that are related to that which should be measured by the test. For example, a questionnaire assessing angina severity would have content validity if the questions centred on the ability to do everyday tasks that made the heart work harder.

Construct validity: The extent to which the test measures a theoretical concept by a specific measuring device or procedure. For example, an IQ test would have construct validity if its results reflected the theoretical concept of intelligence.

Incremental validity: The extent to which the test provides a significant improvement in addition to the use of another approach. A test has incremental validity if it helps more than not using it. For example, ultrasound scanning gives better estimates of fetal gestation age than clinical examination alone.

Scenario 10 revisited

Dr Harrison wrote back to the young researcher, stating that, "Selecting patients and assessing them on the basis of their viewing habits seems inappropriate to me. Hypothyroid patients may do many things apart from increase their television viewing time (and I'm not even sure about that!), so it appears to me that a more valid assessment method is required."

ENDPOINTS

Studies report results in terms of the endpoints that were measured. There are numerous endpoints that can be used in studies; for example, mortality, disease progression, disability, improvement of symptoms in patients and quality of life measures.

Ideally, changes in endpoints should help doctors make better decisions for their patients and have some clinical significance.

There are three main groups to consider when assessing the outcomes of a study.

Clinical endpoint: A measurement of a direct clinical outcome, such as mortality, morbidity and survival.

Surrogate endpoint: A measurement of a physical sign used as a substitute for a clinically meaningful endpoint. Surrogate endpoints are believed to be predictive of important clinical outcomes, although the relationship is not guaranteed. They allow effects to be measured sooner. For example, blood pressure reduction may be used as a surrogate endpoint because hypertension is a risk factor for cerebrovascular and cardiovascular events; for atherosclerosis, cardiovascular mortality or myocardial infarction, angiography or ultrasound imaging can be used.

Surrogate markers are used in Phases 1 and 2 of clinical trials – that is, the early stages of drug development. They may also be used in Phase 3 trials, but there is then careful consideration of how accurately the surrogate marker reflects the clinical outcome in question and whether it will be accurate and reliable. Sample size for studies using surrogate markers can be smaller and the trial does not have to be as long-lasting, because changes in the surrogate responses usually occur before the clinical event occurs.

Composite endpoint: These combine several measurements into a single composite endpoint, using a pre-specified algorithm. This is useful when any one event occurs too infrequently to be an endpoint, and overcomes the problem of insufficient power in a study. The primary endpoint – that is, the health parameter that is measured in all study participants to detect a response to treatment – must be specified. Conclusions about the effectiveness of treatment should focus on this measurement. Secondary endpoints are other parameters that are measured in all study participants to help describe the effect of treatment.

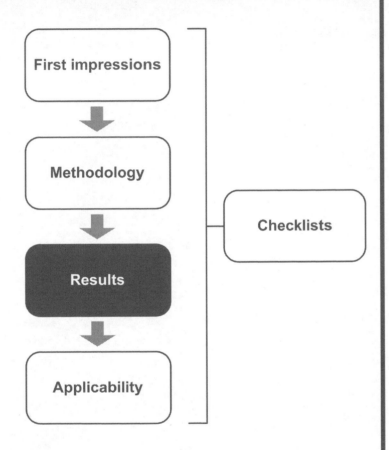

USING STATISTICS

Even the simplest research projects may generate reams of data. Researchers use statistical methods to describe data concisely and make meaningful interpretations of the results.

- Not all statistical methods can be used with all the different data types.
- All the different data types cannot be analysed using just one statistical method.

There are two broad headings to describe the use of statistics:

Descriptive statistics: The use of statistics to describe and summarise observations.

Inferential statistics: The use of statistics to make estimations about the population based on the data collected from the sample population.

The skill in critical appraisal is to understand what data will be generated by the methodology, and to check that the correct statistical method has been applied to the data and that the results are correctly described using the analysis. Only with a valid statistical analysis are the conclusions of a study worth reading.

EPIDEMIOLOGICAL DATA

Epidemiology is the scientific study of the distribution, causes and control of diseases in populations. Studies frequently give epidemiological data to describe the disease or population of interest.

There are two main measures of disease frequency: **incidence** and **prevalence**.

Incidence

Incidence: The rate of occurrence of new cases over a period of time in a defined population.

$$\text{incidence} = \frac{\text{number of new cases over a period of time}}{\text{population size}}$$

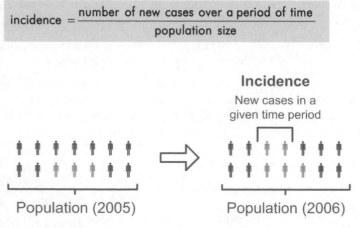

Incidence
New cases in a given time period

Population (2005) → Population (2006)

Figure 16: Incidence

Mortality rate: This is a type of incidence rate that expresses the risk of death over a period of time in a population.

$$\text{mortality rate} = \frac{\text{number of deaths over a period of time}}{\text{population size}}$$

Standardised mortality rate: The mortality rate is adjusted to compensate for a confounder, for example, age.

Standardised mortality ratio: The ratio of the observed standardised mortality rate (from the study population) to the expected standardised mortality rate (from the standard population).

Morbidity rate: This is the rate of occurrence of new non-fatal cases of the disease in a defined population at risk over a given time period.

$$\text{morbidity rate} = \frac{\text{number of new non-fatal cases over a period of time}}{\text{size of population at risk}}$$

Standardised morbidity rate: The morbidity rate is adjusted to compensate for a confounder.

Standardised morbidity ratio: Ratio of the observed standardised morbidity rate (from the study population) to the expected standardised morbidity rate (from the standard population).

Prevalence

Point prevalence: The proportion of a defined population having the disease at a given point in time.

$$\text{point prevalence} = \frac{\text{number of people with the disease at a given time}}{\text{size of population at the same time}}$$

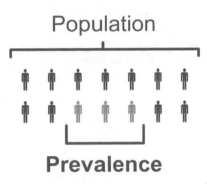

Figure 17: Prevalence

Period prevalence: The proportion of a population that has the disease during a given time period (such as annual prevalence).

$$\text{period prevalence} = \frac{\text{number of people with the disease or developing the disease in a period of time}}{\text{population size during the same period}}$$

Lifetime prevalence: This is the proportion of a population that either has or has had the disease at a given point in time.

Self-assessment exercise 7

1. A cohort study was carried out on 200 men. Half of the participants had been exposed to passive smoking while working in pubs. The other half of the participants had not been exposed to passive smoking. After ten years, there were four cases of lung cancer in the exposed group and one case in the unexposed group. What is the annual incidence rate of lung cancer in the exposed group? What is the annual incidence rate in the unexposed group? What is the overall annual incidence rate?

2. The incidence of cystic fibrosis is one in 2500 births. How many new cases will a paediatrician expect to see over ten years if the hospital she works in delivers 90 babies a month?

3. The annual mortality rate for acute pancreatitis is 1.3 per 100 000. If there are 60 million people in the United Kingdom, how many deaths from acute pancreatitis are expected every week?

4. 85 000 people in the United Kingdom have multiple sclerosis. What is the prevalence rate per 100 000 of the population if the United Kingdom population is 60 million people?

5. What will happen to the prevalence of a disease if there is:

    a. Immigration of cases into the area?
    b. Emigration of cases out of the area?
    c. Immigration of healthy persons into the area?
    d. An increase in the case fatality rate?

UNDERSTANDING THE DATA TYPE

Data can be described as categorical data or quantitative data.

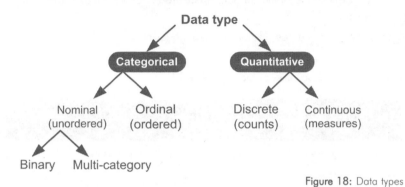

Figure 18: Data types

Categorical data

Data that can be organised into categories are called 'categorical data'.

There are two main groups of categorical data:

1. **Nominal (unordered) data:** There is no inherent order that can be applied to the categories (eg, male or female, dead or alive).
   a. Nominal categorical data can be labelled as **binary** or **dichotomous** data if there are only two categories, such as dead or alive, improved or not improved.
   b. Nominal categorical data can be labelled as **multi-category** if there are more than two categories and the categories have no inherent order, such as married / divorced / engaged / single.
2. **Ordinal (ordered) data:** These differ from nominal data in that they have an inherent order in the categories which is not quantified (eg, the classification grades of a cancer: I, II, III, IV, V). Another example is labelling the severity of an illness as mild, moderate or severe.

Quantitative data

Quantitative data are also known as numerical data and can be subdivided into two groups:

1. **Discrete numerical data (counted):** For example, number of angina attacks in a month.

2. **Continuous numerical data (measured):** For example, body weight.

Quantitative data can be distributed normally or non-normally.

Quantitative data can be converted into categorical data by using cut-off points, particularly for descriptive purposes (**Table 11**).

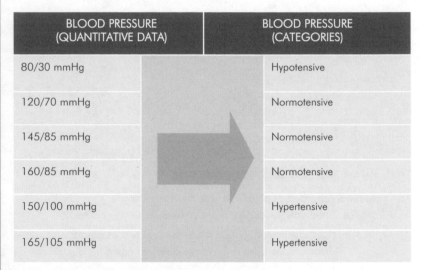

BLOOD PRESSURE (QUANTITATIVE DATA)	BLOOD PRESSURE (CATEGORIES)
80/30 mmHg	Hypotensive
120/70 mmHg	Normotensive
145/85 mmHg	Normotensive
160/85 mmHg	Normotensive
150/100 mmHg	Hypertensive
165/105 mmHg	Hypertensive

Table 11 Converting quantitative data to categorical data

Self-assessment exercise 8

1. What is the data type for each of the variables below?

    a. The diagnosis of patients on a ward.

    b. The sex of patients.

    c. The weight of patients.

    d. The staging of cancer.

    e. The age of patients.

    f. The ethnicity of patients.

    g. The blood cholesterol level.

    h. Patient blood groups.

    i. Body temperature.

    j. Marital status.

    k. Education level.

    l. Number of panic attacks each month.

DESCRIBING DATA FROM ONE SAMPLE

The description of a single set of data should include an indication of the **central tendency** of that data set and a measure of the **spread** of the data around this central tendency. The choice of statistical tests to use to describe a single set of data is dependent upon the type of data collected.

Categorical data (mode, frequency)

Mode: The most common value.

Frequency: The number of values in each category.

For example, from **Table 11**:

> the mode is 'normotensive'
> the frequency is:
> > hypotensive (1 observation)
> > normotensive (3 observations)
> > hypertensive (2 observations)

Non-normally distributed data (median, range, interquartile range)

As shown in **Figure 19**, in non-normally distributed data, the data values are distributed asymmetrically across the distribution.

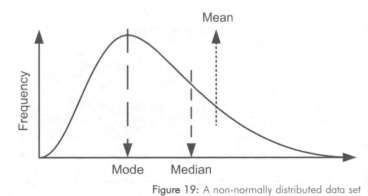

Figure 19: A non-normally distributed data set

Median: From the Latin for 'middle', the median represents the middle value of ordered data observations. With an even number of data values, the median is the average of the two values that lie on either side of the middle place.

The advantages of the median estimation is that it is robust to outliers; that is, it is not affected by aberrant points (unlike the mean). The main disadvantage of using the median is that it does not use all the data in its determination.

Range: This is the difference between the lowest and highest values in the data set. It is useful for skewed data but it is not robust to aberrant values.

DATA SET	MEDIAN	RANGE
1, 2, 3, 3, 5	middle value is 3	5 – 1 = 4
1, 2, 3, 3, 5, 7, 8, 10	(3 + 5) /2 = 4/	10 – 1 = 9

Table 12 Example calculations of median and range

Interquartile range: This is a 'mini' range because it focuses on the spread of the middle 50% of the data. It is usually reported alongside the median value of the data set.

The data are ranked in order and divided into four equal parts (irrespective of their values). The points at 25%, 50% and 75% of the distribution are identified. These are known as the quartiles and the median is the second quartile. The interquartile range is between the 1st and 3rd quartiles (**Figure 20**).

Unlike the range, the interquartile range is not influenced by outliers and is relatively easy to calculate. However, the interquartile range does not incorporate all the presented values.

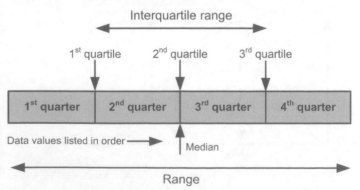

Figure 20: Comparing the range and the interquartile range

If the number of data values is not divisible by four, first identify the median value and then calculate the 1st and 3rd quartiles by the middle values between the median and the end of the ranges.

Normally distributed data (mean, standard deviation)

A normal distribution, also known as a Gaussian distribution, is a perfectly symmetric bell-shaped curve, as shown in **Figure 21**.

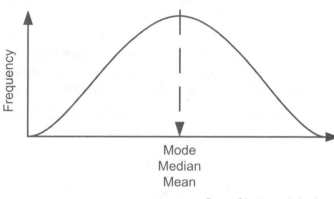

Mode
Median
Mean

Figure 21: Normal distribution

Mean: The sum of all the values divided by the number of values:

$$\text{mean} = \frac{\text{sum of all the values}}{\text{the number of values}} \qquad \bar{x} = \sum \frac{x}{n}$$

The mean uses all the data and is easy to calculate; however, it is still not robust to aberrant values and can be difficult to interpret.

In a perfect normal distribution, the mean, median and mode are of equal value and lie in the centre of the distribution.

Standard deviation (SD): A statistical measure that describes the degree of data spread about the mean – the amount the values will deviate from the mean.

Standard deviation is calculated as the square root of the variance. The variance is the sum of all the differences between all the values and the mean, squared, and divided by the total number of observations minus 1 (the degrees of freedom).

$$\text{standard deviation} = \sqrt{v} = \sqrt{\frac{\sum (x - \bar{x})^2}{n - 1}}$$

The extent of the bell shape in a normal distribution is dependent upon the standard deviation. Key properties of the normal distribution are that we can calculate the proportion of the observations that will lie between any two values of the variable as long as we know the mean and standard deviation.

If observations follow a normal distribution, the standard deviation is a useful measure of the spread of these observations.

- A range covered by 1 SD above the mean and 1 SD below the mean includes 68% of the observations (ie, the area under the curve) (Figure 22).
- A range of 2 SDs (actually 1.96) above and below the mean includes about 95% of the observations (**Figure 23**).
- A range of 3 SDs (actually 2.58) above and below the mean includes 99.7% of the observations (**Figure 24**).

In a non-normally distributed population (skewed), the mean will be a biased estimate of the centre of the data; for example, duration of stay in hospital.

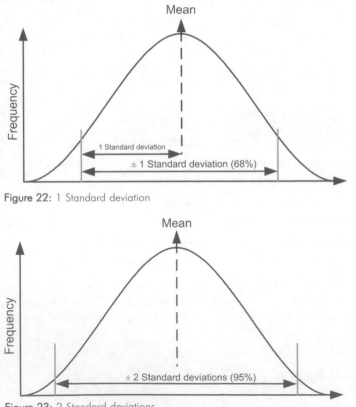

Figure 22: 1 Standard deviation

Figure 23: 2 Standard deviations

THE DOCTOR'S GUIDE TO CRITICAL APPRAISAL

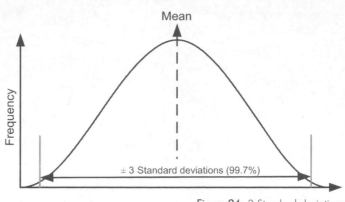

Figure 24: 3 Standard deviations

The larger the standard deviation, the greater the spread of observations around the mean (**Figure 25**).

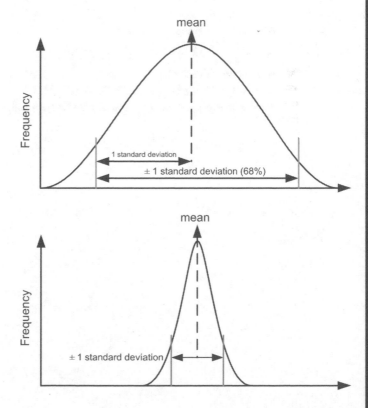

Figure 25: Large standard deviation (top) compared with small standard deviation (bottom)

Self-assessment exercise 9

1. In this data set: 1, 2, 2, 3, 3, 3, 4, 4, 5
   - a. What is the mode?
   - b. What is the frequency?
   - c. What is the median?
   - d. What is the range?
   - e. What is the mean?

2. In this data set: 5, 10, 15, 20, 100
   - a. What is the median?
   - b. What is the range?
   - c. What is the mean?
   - d. Which describes the central tendency of this data set better – the median or the mean?

3. In this data set: 5, 10, 15, 20, 25, 30, 35, 40, 45, 50, 60, 70
   - a. What is the median?
   - b. What is the range?
   - c. What is the interquartile range?

4. In this data set: 3, 13, 44, 45, 51, 56, 66, 75, 91, 102
   - a. What is the mean?
   - b. What is the standard deviation?
   - c. What is the range in which 95% of observations will lie?

INFERRING POPULATION RESULTS FROM SAMPLES

To generalise the result from a random sample to the target population, two concepts need to be understood:

- standard error
- confidence intervals

Standard error (SE)

Suppose that an experiment is set up to measure the mean height of the population. A random sample of the population will be selected to take part in the study. The results from the sample will be generalised to the population.

If the study is repeated with a new random sample, the mean height from this new sample may not be the same as that from the first random sample. Indeed, repeating the study several times may produce a series of different mean heights. This is shown in **Table 13**.

	MEAN HEIGHT	STANDARD DEVIATION
Sample 1	1.65	0.12
Sample 2	1.58	0.23
Sample 3	1.63	0.19
Sample 4	1.88	0.22
Sample 5	1.59	0.18
Sample 6	1.44	0.20
Sample 7	1.63	0.05
Sample 8	1.49	0.14

Table 13 Mean heights and standard deviations from different samples

If these sample means are themselves plotted on a graph, they too will follow a normal distribution with their own mean and standard deviation. The standard deviation of the sample means has its own name: **standard error**.

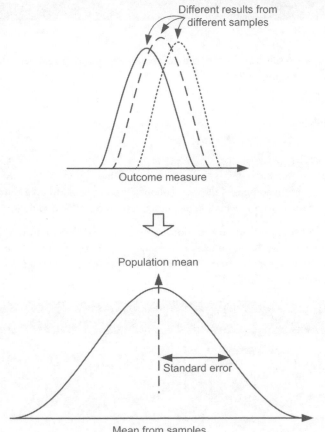

Figure 26: Population mean and standard error

$$\text{standard error of a sample of sample size } n = \frac{\text{standard deviation}}{\sqrt{n}}$$

n = number of observations in the sample

The more observations you have, the smaller will be the standard error – that is, the more likely the sample mean ($\bar{x}$) reflects the true mean value (μ) of a parameter in the general population.

Confidence intervals

Suppose we wish to measure the mean height of children in a school. There may be too many children to measure, so we may take a sample. We may, for example, measure the heights of 20 children chosen at random during the lunch break.

If we measure the height of one child, we can be very sure the result reflects the child's height (validity and reliability). If we measure all the children, we can get a mean height for the 20 children. To generalise this to the whole school, we need to be able to express the certainty with which we estimate the mean height to be correct.

Confidence intervals measure the uncertainty in measurements. They can be described as a range of values which, when quoted in relation to an estimate, express the degree of uncertainty around that estimate. The width of the confidence interval indicates the precision of the estimate. The 95% confidence interval is routinely quoted; it is the range within which we can be 95% confident that the true value for the population lies.

We can make a wide estimate with a high degree of confidence or a more precise estimate with a lower degree of confidence. The larger the sample, the less variable the observations are, the more likely the results are to be true – that is, the narrower the confidence interval, the more confidence one can have in making inferences about the population parameters.

95% confidence interval for a population mean =
mean ± 1.96 × standard error

- When quoted alongside a difference between two groups (eg, mean difference), a confidence interval that includes 0 is statistically non-significant.

- When quoted alongside a ratio (eg, relative risk, odds ratio, etc.), a confidence interval that includes 1 is statistically non-significant.

Self-assessment exercise 10

1. In this data set: 10, 12, 15, 17, 18, 19, 21

   a. What is the mean?
   b. What is the median?
   c. What is the standard deviation?
   d. What is the standard error?

2. In this data set: 10, 12, 15, 17, 18, 19, 91

   a. What is the mean?
   b. What is the median?
   c. What is the standard deviation?
   d. What is the standard error?

COMPARING SAMPLES – THE NULL HYPOTHESIS

Often in research, the results from two or more samples are compared. The researcher is interested in finding out if there are any differences between the groups, as they may highlight an important role for an exposure, investigation or treatment.

To complicate matters, by convention this task is turned on its head, with the researcher assuming that any differences seen are due to chance. The researcher then calculates how likely such differences are indeed due to chance, hoping to show that it, is in fact, very unlikely.

Step one – the null hypothesis
The **null hypothesis** states that any difference observed in the results of two or more groups is due to chance.

> The null hypothesis is rarely stated in clinical papers and should not be confused with the primary hypothesis. The importance of the null hypothesis lies in the fact that it underpins the statistical tests.

For example, the initial research question may be, 'Does a relationship exist between cannabis smoking and the development of schizophrenia?' The researcher may set up a case–control study to look at past cannabis smoking in a group of schizophrenic patients and matched controls. If there are differences in the exposure to cannabis smoking between the two groups, the researcher expresses this difference in terms of the null hypothesis, such as 'no relationship exists between cannabis use and schizophrenia.' The researcher then uses statistical tests to calculate the probability that the difference is indeed due to chance and decide whether this probability is large enough to accept, in which case the null hypothesis stands true.

If the results are unlikely to be explained by chance alone, the null hypothesis is rejected and the **alternative hypothesis**, which states that there is a difference not due to chance, is accepted.

Step two – calculating probabilities
Probability is the likelihood of any event occurring as a proportion of the total number of possibilities. The probability of an event varies between 0.0 (never happens) to 1.0 (certain to happen).

Probability in clinical papers is often expressed as the '**P value**'. *P* values express the probability of getting the observed results given a true null hypothesis. *P* values are calculated using statistical methods.

$P < 0.05$ means that the probability of obtaining a given result by chance is less than one in 20. By convention, a *P* value of less than 0.05 is the accepted threshold for **statistical significance** – that is, the null hypothesis can be rejected.

P values greater than 0.05 are non-significant – that is, the null hypothesis is accepted.

This is summarised in **Table 14**. **Table 15** explains the roles of probability in rejecting the null hypothesis in another way. *P* values may be calculated by several statistical techniques.

$P < 0.05$	$P \geq 0.05$
Less than 1 in 20	Greater than or equal to 1 in 20
Results significant	Results non-significant
Null hypothesis is rejected	Null hypothesis is accepted
Evidence of association between variable and outcome	Unproven association between variable and outcome

Table 14 Understanding *P* values and significance

EVENT	WHAT OTHER PEOPLE SAY	WHAT A RESEARCHER SAYS
Week 1 Dr Cash wins £5 million pounds on the National Lottery	He is as likely as anyone else to win the lottery. His win was due to chance	Null hypothesis: Dr Cash is no more likely to win the lottery than anyone else. The null hypothesis holds true
Week 2 Dr Cash wins the National Lottery again	He is as likely to win as anyone else, even though he won it last week too. He's just incredibly lucky	Null hypothesis: Dr Cash is no more likely to win the lottery than anyone else. The probability of him winning twice in two weeks is even more unlikely, but it can happen. The null hypothesis holds true
Week 3 Dr Cash wins the National Lottery for the third week in a row	We suspect Dr Cash has not won the lottery three times simply by chance. There is something else going on here to explain these events	The null hypothesis is rejected: the association between Dr Cash and the three consecutive lottery wins is not due simply to chance. The probability of this happening is so small that it is not acceptable

Table 15 The role of probability in rejecting the null hypothesis

Step 3 – type 1 and type 2 errors

Type 1 errors

A type 1 error occurs when the null hypothesis is rejected when it is true. A **false positive** result has been recorded because a difference is found between groups when no such difference exists. Type 1 errors are usually attributable to bias and/or confounding factors.

If a difference is seen between two groups, a type 1 error can be avoided by significance testing. P values should be quoted alongside the results. $P = 0.05$ is used as the level of risk we are prepared to take that we will make a type 1 error. The probability of making a type 1 error is equal to P and expressed as α. For example $\alpha = 0.05$ means that there is only a 5% chance of erroneously rejecting the null hypothesis.

Type 2 errors

A type 2 error occurs when the null hypothesis is accepted when it is in fact false. The study has returned a **false negative** result after failing to uncover a difference between the groups that actually exists. This usually happens because the sample size is not large enough and/or the measurement variance is too large.

Type 2 errors can be avoided at the design stage of the study by power calculations that give an indication of how many participants are required in the trial to minimise type 2 errors. The probability of making a type 2 error is represented by ß.

Figure 27 and **Table 16** summarise the discussion so far.

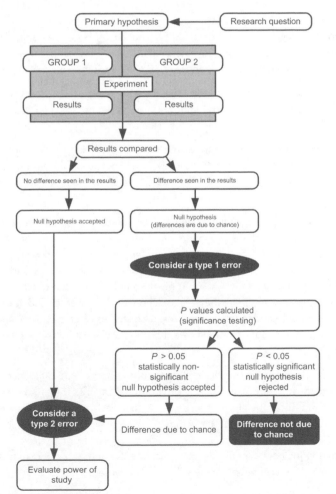

Figure 27: The null hypothesis, P values and type 1 and 2 errors

		NULL HYPOTHESIS	
		True	False
EXPERIMENTAL RESULT	Significant	Type 1 error	Correct
	Not significant	Correct	Type 2 error

Table 16 Summary of type 1 and 2 errors

Sample size and power

The **sample size** for a study is not simply chosen at random. Ideally, a clinical trial should be large enough to detect reliably the smallest possible difference in the outcome measure, with treatment, that is considered clinically worthwhile.

The **power** of a study is its ability to detect a true difference in outcome between the control arm and the intervention arm. This is defined as the probability that a type 2 error will not be made in that study.

Power calculations are made to ensure that the study is large enough to have a high chance of detecting a statistically significant result if one truly did exist. As a general rule, the larger the sample size of a study the more power the study is said to have.

It is not uncommon for studies to be underpowered, failing to detect even large treatment effects because of inadequate sample size. A calculation should be performed at the start of a study to determine the degree of power chosen for that study. For example, a power of 0.8 means there is an 80% probability of finding a significant difference with a given sample size, if a real difference truly did exist, having excluded the role of chance. **A power of 0.8 is generally accepted as being adequate in most research studies**. A study power set at 80% accepts a likelihood of one in five (that is, 20%) of missing such a real difference.

The probability of rejecting the null hypothesis when a true difference exists is represented as $1 - \beta$. Typically, β is arbitrarily set at 0.2. Therefore a study has 80% power (0.8 of a chance) to detect a specified degree of difference at a specified degree of significance. A power calculation is used to determine the number of patients required before a difference in response between groups becomes significant – that is, we can calculate the numbers of patients required to minimise the likelihood of a type 2 error occurring.

The key is to power the study adequately. Sometimes studies are double checked by performing an interim analysis.

One-tailed versus two-tailed significance tests

The **alternative hypothesis** is the proposed experimental hypothesis that runs opposite to the null hypothesis.

One-tailed significance tests are used to examine only one direction of the alternative hypothesis, disregarding the opposite direction.

Alternatively, two-tailed significance tests are significance tests that make no assumptions about the direction of difference and examine both directions. Two-tailed tests are performed when there is no expectation about the difference.

For example, if you were comparing the population means of two groups of patients, a one-tailed test considers as an alternative hypothesis that the mean of sample A is greater than the mean of sample B. A two-tailed test would consider as an alternative hypothesis that the mean of sample A is either greater or less than that of sample B (Figure 28).

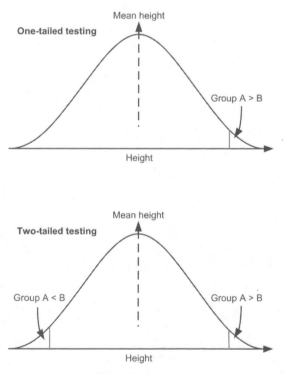

Figure 28: One-tailed and two-tailed tests

Clinical significance

Statistical significance as shown by *P* values is not the same as clinical significance. Statistical significance judges whether treatment effects are explicable as chance findings. Clinical significance assesses whether treatment effects are worthwhile in real life. Small improvements that are statistically significant may not result in any meaningful improvement clinically.

Self-assessment exercise 11

How would you write the following clinical questions in terms of the null hypothesis?

1. Do patients have problems when they stop paroxetine suddenly?

2. Is atorvastatin more effective than simvastatin at lowering cholesterol levels?

COMPARING SAMPLES – STATISTICAL TESTS

Samples are compared using a variety of statistical tests. Not all statistical tests can be used with all data sets. The determining factors are the number of samples we are comparing, the type of data in the samples and whether the data are paired or unpaired.

The term 'unpaired' ('independent') data refers to two groups having different members. Here the selection of the individuals for one group must not be influenced by or related to the selection of the other group. 'Paired' data refers to data for the same individuals at different time points.

Table 17 summarises the statistical tests to use.

	CATEGORICAL DATA	NON-PARAMET-RIC DATA	PARAMETRIC DATA
ONE SAMPLE	Chi-squared test Fisher's exact test (small sample)	Wilcoxon signed rank test	One-sample *t*-test
COMPARING TWO GROUPS	Chi-squared test (unpaired) McNemar's test (paired)	Mann–Whitney *U* test (unpaired) Wilcoxon rank sum test (paired)	*t*-test (paired or unpaired)
COMPARING MORE THAN TWO GROUPS	Chi-squared test (unpaired) McNemar's test (paired)	Kruskal–Wallis ANOVA (unpaired) Friedman test (paired)	ANOVA (paired or unpaired)

ANOVA = ANALYSIS OF VARIANCE

Table 17 A summary of statistical tests for comparing samples

Categorical data

Categorical statistical tests involve the use of **contingency tables**, also known as **2 × 2 tables** (**Table 18**). The contingency table consists of rows and columns of cells. The frequencies of the events are recorded in the relevant boxes. Contingency tables can be a source of confusion, because there are different ways of displaying the same information. Always maintain a consistent approach by having the exposure factor or intervention across the rows and the disease status or outcome status down the columns.

		Disease status / outcome status		
		positive	negative	Totals
Exposure to risk / treatment / interventions / test results	positive	a	b	a + b
	negative	c	d	c + d
	Totals	a + c	b + d	a + b + c + d

Table 18 The format of a 2 × 2 table

The statistical tests used with categorical data are the Chi-squared (χ^2) test (unpaired data) and McNemar's test (paired binary data). For small-sized samples (fewer than five observations in any cell), the Fisher's exact test can be used (**Figure 29**).

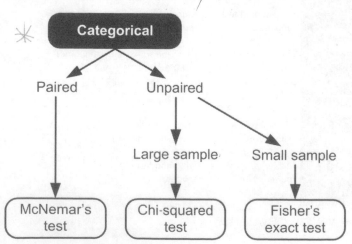

Figure 29: The statistical tests used with categorical data

Degrees of freedom: This is an estimate of the number of independent categories in a particular statistical test or experiment. Dependent categories can be calculated from the independent categories. In the case of a 2×2 contingency table, it is the number of ways in which the results in the table can vary, given the column and row totals. A 2×2 table has two columns and two rows. If the result in one of the row cells is changed, the result in the other row cell can be calculated. Similarly, if the result in one of the column cells is changed, the result in the other column cell can be calculated.

Thus degrees of freedom is [(rows minus 1) multiplied by (columns minus 1)].

Continuous data

Parametric tests are used for data that are normally distributed. These include the *t*-test and analysis of variance (ANOVA).

Non-normally distributed data can either be mathematically transformed into a normal-like distribution by taking powers, reciprocals or logarithms of data values or, alternatively, statistical tests may be used that don't have the assumption of normality.

Non-parametric tests, also referred to as 'distribution-free statistics', are used for analysis of non-normally distributed data. The most commonly used tests are, for two groups: the Mann–Whitney *U* test (unpaired groups), Wilcoxon's rank sum test (for paired data) and, for two or more groups: the Kruskal–Wallis ANOVA (for unpaired data) and the Friedman test (paired data) (**Figure 30**).

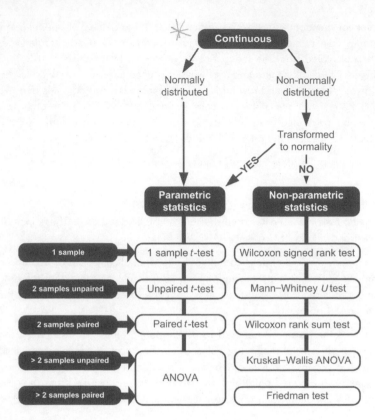

Figure 30: The statistical tests used with continuous data

COMPARING RELATIONSHIPS BETWEEN VARIABLES

So far, we have described the data from a single sample, inferred population data from data samples, and compared samples using the null hypothesis. Sometimes it is necessary to establish the nature of the relationship between two or more variables to see if they are associated.

Multivariate statistics enable us to examine the relationships between several variables and make predictions about the data set. There are several methods, depending on the number of variables being examined.

Continuous data can be analysed using correlation and regression techniques.

Correlation

Correlation assesses the **strength** of the relationship between two quantitative variables (**Figure 31**). It examines whether a linear association exists between two variables, X and Y. X is usually the independent variable and Y is usually the dependent variable.

- A **positive correlation** means that Y increases linearly as X increases.

- A **negative correlation** means that Y decreases linearly as X increases.

- **Zero correlation** reflects a complete non-association between the compared variables.

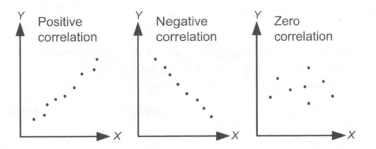

Figure 31: Three types of correlation

Correlation coefficient

The magnitude and direction of any identified linear association is expressed as a **correlation coefficient**, with a P value and confidence intervals. The P value indicates whether the association could have arisen by chance. If $P < 0.05$, then the coefficient has a significant influence on the dependent variable in that population and the association did not arise by chance. The correlation coefficient ranges from -1 to $+1$.

The correlation coefficient only tells you if there is an **association** between the variables, not whether the relationship is causal.

There are three types of correlation coefficient, depending on the types of data being compared.

1. **Pearson's correlation coefficient, r**

   This is a parametric correlation coefficient used to measure the association between continuous variables that are both normally distributed.

   r^2 is the 'coefficient of determination' – an estimate of the percent variation in one variable that is explained by the other variable.

2. **Spearman's rank correlation coefficient, ρ (rho)**

   Used for two ordinal variables or when one variable has a continuous normal distribution and the other is categorical or non-normally distributed.

3. **Kendall's correlation coefficient, τ (tau)**

   For correlation between two categorical or non-normally distributed variables.

Regression

Regression determines the nature of the relationship between two or more variables. It involves estimating the best straight line to summarise the association.

The **regression equation** indicates how much Y changes with any given change in X. The equation enables Y to be **predicted** from X. The precision of this estimate depends upon the degree of correlation.

The regression equation can be used to construct a regression line or scatter diagram. It does not prove causality.

Simple linear regression

Where there is one independent variable, the equation of the best fit for the regression line is:

$$Y = a + bX$$

(**Figure 32**).

Y = value of the outcome variable.

a = intercept of the regression line on the y axis.

b = regression coefficient (slope of the regression line), describing the strength of the relationship.

X = value of the independent variable.

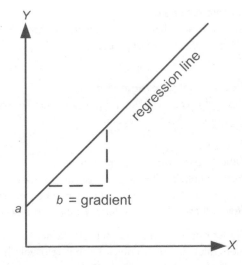

Figure 32: Simple linear regression

For a given value of X, a corresponding value of Y can be predicted.

Multiple linear regression

A regression model in which the dependent outcome variable is predicted from two or more independent variables is called 'multiple linear regression'. The independent variables may be continuous or categorical.

A measure of association is calculated taking a number of variables into account simultaneously:

$$Y = a + b_1X_1 + b_2X_2 + \ldots$$

$a = Y$ when all the independent variables are zero.

$b_1, b_2, \ldots$ = partial regression coefficients for each independent variable. These are calculated by the **least squares method**. This is usually presented along with a 95% confidence interval and a P value. If $P < 0.05$ or the confidence interval does not contain zero, then the independent variable has a significant influence on the dependent variable.

Multiple linear regression is used to assess what effect different variables may have on the study outcome. It is also used to assess the effects of possible confounding factors that may be present in the study.

Logistic regression

This is used where the outcome variable Y is binary in nature and the independents are of any type.

Proportional Cox regression

This is also known as the 'proportional hazards regression' and is used to assess survival or other time-related event.

Other types of multivariate statistics

Factor analysis: This is a statistical approach that can be used to analyse interrelationships among a large number of variables and can be used to explain these variables in terms of their common underlying factors.

Cluster analysis: This is a multivariate analysis technique that tries to organise information about variables so that relatively homogeneous groups, clusters, can be formed.

The **analysis of variance test (ANOVA)** also has some multivariate extensions:

- **ANCOVA (analysis of covariance):** This is similar to multiple regression.
- **MANOVA (multiple analysis of variance):** This is used with multiple dependent variables and useful for multiple hypothesis testing.
- **MANCOVA (multiple analysis of covariance):** This is used with multiple dependent and independent variables.

RISKS AND ODDS

Describing risk in a group
Risk and odds apply to a single group of people.

Risk: In clinical research, risk has the same meaning as probability. Risk is the probability of something happening. Risk is the number of times an event is likely to occur divided by the total number of events possible. It is expressed as P and is presented either as a number between 0 and 1 or as a percentage.

Odds: Odds is also another way of expressing chance. The odds is the ratio of the number of times an event is likely to occur divided by the number of times it is likely not to occur. This is expressed as a ratio or fraction.

For example, if someone is expecting a baby:

- the risk of it being a girl is ½ – that is, 50%
- the odds of it being a girl is 1/1 = 1 – that is, it is as likely to be a girl as it is not to be a girl.

Comparing risk between groups
If two groups are being compared, relative risk and odds ratio compare the two groups with respect to the likelihood of an event occurring, and describe the risk of people having an outcome in the presence of an exposure.

2 × 2 contingency tables
The most common way to calculate the risk ratio is to start with tabulating the results in a 2 × 2 table, where each cell in the table contains the number of participants in each category (**Table 19**). This ensures all the calculations are performed in a consistent way.

		Disease status / outcome status		
		positive	negative	Totals
Exposure to risk / treatment / interventions	positive	a	b	a + b
	negative	c	d	c + d
	Totals	a + c	b + d	a + b + c + d

Table 19 2 × 2 Contingency table

Other aspects of risk can be derived from the 2 × 2 contingency table (**Table 20**).

	FORMULA
Control Event Rate (CER) (outcome event rate in control group)	$\dfrac{c}{c + d}$
Experimental Event Rate (EER) (outcome event rate in experimental group)	$\dfrac{a}{a + b}$
Absolute Risk Reduction (ARR)	$CER - \cancel{AAR}\ EER$
Relative Risk (RR)	$\dfrac{EER}{CER}$
Relative Risk Reduction (RRR)	$\dfrac{CER - EER}{CER}$
Number Needed to Treat (NNT)	$\dfrac{1}{ARR}$
Odds of outcome in exposed group	$\dfrac{a}{b}$
Odds of outcome in non-exposed group	$\dfrac{c}{d}$
Odds ratio (OR)	$\dfrac{a / b}{c / d} = \dfrac{ad}{bc}$

Table 20 Derivation of other aspects of risk from the 2 × 2 contingency table

Absolute risk

The incidence rate of the outcome in the group (which can be the treated or the untreated population).

$$Control\ event\ rate\ (CER) = \frac{c}{c + d}$$

$$Experimental\ event\ rate\ (EER) = \frac{a}{a + b}$$

Absolute risk reduction

Absolute risk reduction (ARR) is the absolute risk in the untreated group minus the absolute risk in the treated group:

$$Absolute\ risk\ reduction = CER - EER$$

Relative risk

Relative risk (RR) or risk ratio is the absolute risk in the experimental group divided by the absolute risk in the control group:

$$Relative\ risk = \frac{EER}{CER}$$

- If the relative risk is statistically significant different from 1, there is evidence of an **association**.
- If the relative risk is equal to 1, there is **no risk difference** between the groups.
- If the relative risk is greater than 1, there is an **increased risk** amongst those exposed to the factor.
- If the relative risk is less than 1, the factor is **protective** against the disease.

Relative risk reduction

Relative risk reduction (RRR) is the proportional reduction in rates of bad outcomes between treated and control patients in a study.

$$Relative\ risk\ reduction = \frac{CER - EER}{CER}$$

Number needed to treat

The number needed to treat (NNT) is the number of patients that must be treated with the intervention, compared with the control, for one patient to experience the beneficial effect. It is the reciprocal of the absolute risk reduction between two interventions. It can also be used to assess adverse events (**number needed to harm**). The nearer the number needed to treat is to '1', the better. Comparisons between numbers needed to treat can only be made if the baseline risks are the same.

$$Number\ needed\ to\ treat = \frac{1}{ARR}$$

Odds ratio

Odds ratio (OR) is an alternative way of comparing how 'likely' events are between two groups.

Odds ratio is the ratio of the odds of having the disorder in the experimental group relative to the odds in favour of having the disorder in the control group.

It is used in cross-sectional studies and case–control studies. In a case–control study, the exposure is often the presence or absence of a risk factor for a disease, and the outcome is the presence or absence of the disease.

$$Odds\ ratio\ =\ \frac{ad}{bc}$$

- An odds ratio of 1.0 (or unity) reflects exactly the same outcome rates in both groups – that is, **no effect**.

- An odds ratio greater than 1 indicates that the estimated **likelihood** of developing disease is **greater** in the exposed than in the unexposed group.

- An odds ratio less than one indicates that the estimated **likelihood** of developing the disease is **less** in the exposed than in the unexposed group.

Self-assessment exercise 12

1. In a group of 60 patients treated with diclofenac sodium, 10 complained of indigestion. What are the risk and odds of developing this side-effect in this group?

2. In a group of 220 patients with heart disease, the risk of death in the first year is 5%. How many patients will die in the first year?

3. In a cohort study, 100 patients were followed up for 20 years. At the start, 56 of the patients had been exposed to asbestos. At the end of the study, of those exposed to asbestos, 20 had lung disease. Of those not exposed, only 2 had lung disease. Tabulate this information in a contingency table. Calculate the control event rate (CER) and the experimental event rate (EER). Calculate the odds of the outcome in the exposed group and the odds of the outcome in the non-exposed group.

4. 2000 patients with fungal nail infections were randomly allocated to a new topical treatment or placebo (in equal numbers). 66 patients in the placebo group had another infection within 1 month, compared with 21 patients in the treated group. Draw a 2 × 2 table for this information and calculate the following: absolute risk in the treated group (EER), absolute risk in the untreated group (CER), the relative risk (RR), the relative risk reduction (RRR), the absolute risk reduction (ARR) and the number needed to treat (NNT).

5. In a case–control study, 17 patients treated with a new analgesic reported a significant improvement in pain symptoms, whereas 4 patients did not. In a control group treated with paracetamol, only 1 of the 20 patients reported a benefit. Calculate the control event rate (CER), the experimental event rate (EER) and the odds ratio (OR).

6. If the relative risk is 1.8 with a 95% confidence interval of 0.7 to 2.1, what does this mean?

SYSTEMATIC REVIEWS AND META-ANALYSES

So far, we have been critically appraising individual studies. However, a literature search often reveals many studies with similar aims and hypotheses. Examining one study in isolation may mean that we miss out on findings discovered by other researchers. Ideally, all the studies around one subject area should be collated.

Reviews of articles provide a useful summary of the literature in a particular field. The main flaw with many of these reviews is that they are based on a selection of papers collected in a non-systematic way, so that important research may have been missed.

A **systematic review** attempts to access and review systematically all of the pertinent articles in the field. A systematic review should effectively explain the research question, the search strategy and the designs of the studies that were selected. The results of these studies are then pooled and as a result the evidence drawn from systematic reviews can be very powerful and valuable. The overall conclusions are more accurate and reliable than individual studies. Systematic reviews are the gold-standard source of research evidence in the hierarchy of research evidence.

There are four key components to systematic reviews (**Table 21**).

Specifying the research question	Pre-specification of study types Subjects, inclusion, exclusions Intervention / exposure Outcomes Statistical methods
Search strategy	Reproducible Comprehensive Unbiased
Extracting the data	Standardised proforma Study methodology details Assessment of study quality
Interpretation of data	Fixed or random effects models Publication bias for small negative studies Heterogeneity

Table 21 Components of systematic reviews

The QUOROM statement

A conference referred to as the Quality Of Reporting Of Meta-analyses (QUOROM) was held to improve the quality of systematic reviews. This conference resulted in the creation of the QUOROM Statement, which consists of a flow diagram and a checklist of 18 items covering the abstract, introduction, methods and results section of a report of a systematic review of randomised trials[8]. The checklist encourages authors to provide readers with information regarding how the review was set up. The flow diagram provides information about the progress of randomised trials throughout the review process, from the number of potentially relevant trials identified to those retrieved and ultimately included.

Meta-analysis

A meta-analysis combines the results of several studies. Meta-analyses are performed when more than one study has estimated the effect of an intervention and when there are no differences in participants, interventions and settings that are likely to affect the outcome significantly. It is also important that the outcome in the different trials has been measured in similar ways.

The results from the studies that have been conducted on a specific clinical question are combined to produce an overall estimate of effect, which will include all the information that has been provided by all the studies.

A good meta-analysis is based on a systematic review of studies and not from a non-systematic review. A non-systematic review can introduce bias into the analysis.

The key steps to remember for a meta-analysis are:

- Synthesis using statistical techniques to combine results of included studies.
- Calculation of a pooled estimate of effect of an intervention together with its *P* value and confidence interval.
- Check for variations between the studies (heterogeneity).
- Check for publication bias.
- Review and interpret the findings.

8 Moher D, Cook DJ, Eastwood S, Olkin I, Rennie D, Stroup DF, for the QUOROM Group. Improving the quality of reports of meta-analyses of randomised controlled trials: the QUOROM statement. *Lancet*, 1999, 354, 1896–900.

Forest plots

The results of a meta-analysis are presented as a forest plot or blobbogram of pooled results.

The forest plot is a diagram with a list of studies on the vertical axis, often arranged in order of effect or chronological order, and the common outcome measure on the horizontal axis. The outcome measure may be odds or risk ratio, means, event rates, etc. There is a vertical 'line of no effect', which intersects the horizontal axis at the point that signifies there is no difference between the interventions.

The result of each study is shown by a box that represents the point estimate of the outcome measure. The area of the box is proportional to the weight each study is given in the meta-analysis. Studies with larger samples sizes are given weight, as are studies with more precise estimates (ie, tighter confidence intervals).

Across each box there is a horizontal line. The width of the horizontal line represents the 95% confidence interval.

If the horizontal line touches or crosses the line of no effect, either the study outcome is not statistically significant and/or the sample size was too small to allow us to be confident about where the true result lies.

If the horizontal line does not cross the line of unity, the results are statistically significant.

The overall outcome of the meta-analysis is a diamond shape. The position of the widest part of the diamond is located at the point estimate of the pooled result. The horizontal width of the diamond is the 95% confidence interval.

Figure 33 summarises the components of a forest plot.

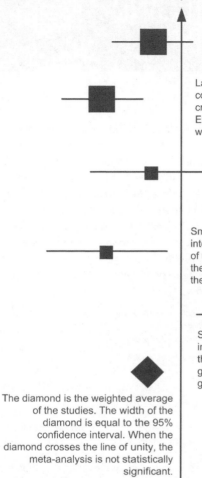
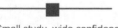

Figure 33: Understanding a forest plot

Did you know?

The Cochrane Collaboration logo illustrates a forest plot from a systematic review of randomised controlled trials of corticosteroid treatment given to women about to go into premature labour. The forest plot indicates that corticosteroids reduce the risk of babies dying from the complications of immaturity.

HETEROGENEITY AND HOMOGENEITY

Scenario 11

A randomised controlled trial comparing antidepressant treatment against placebo took place in three centres: Manchester, Birmingham and London. The results for Manchester and London were similar. The patients in Birmingham reported remarkably different results, with much bigger improvements in depressive rating scale scores. Before the results of the three centres were combined, a scrutiny of the methodology used in each centre indicated a methodological difference. In Manchester and London, patients were invited to busy outpatient departments to report their progress. In Birmingham, the patients were invited to a hotel suite where they were given tea and cakes while waiting for the researchers. The researchers commented that the difference in results was not due to random chance alone.

Because the aim of the meta-analysis is to summate the results of similar studies, there are tests to ensure that the studies merit combination. Any variation seen to occur between study results can be due to chance or systematic differences or both.

Homogeneity is said to occur when studies have similar and consistent results and any observed differences are due to random variation.

When there is more variation than would be expected by chance alone, even after allowing for random variation, this is referred to as **heterogeneity**.

If there is substantial heterogeneity between studies, this can bias the summary effect and the summary statistic is therefore unreliable. By identifying heterogeneity, you can adjust and correct the overall results before producing an overall estimate.

Heterogeneity can occur at different stages. It can occur as differences in the composition of the groups, in the design of the study and in the outcome; for example, differences in population characteristics, baseline risks, prescribing effects, clinical settings, methodological differences, outcome measures and, sometimes, unknown differences. It can also occur if the studies are small and the event rate is low so that the results for the groups differ significantly and you cannot rely on the summary estimate.

Clinical heterogeneity occurs when the individuals chosen for two studies differ from one another significantly, making the results of these studies difficult to collate.

Statistical heterogeneity occurs when the results of the different studies differ from one another significantly more than would be expected by chance.

Summary effect size

There are two ways to calculate the effect size to summarise the results for a meta-analysis.

1. **Fixed-effects model:** This assumes that there is no heterogeneity between the studies – that is, the trials are all comparable and any differences that may be present are due to the treatments themselves (homogeneity).

2. **Random-effects model:** This allows for between-study variations when the pooled overall effect estimate is produced (heterogeneity).

If heterogeneity has been ruled out, a fixed-effects model is used. If heterogeneity does exist, a random-effects model is used.

The two types of fixed-effects models for relative risk and odds ratio used to produce a summary statistic are:

1. **The Mantel–Haenszel procedure:** The most widely used statistical method for producing the final result of a forest plot. It combines the results of trials, to produce a single-value overall summary of the net effect. The result is given as a Chi-squared statistic associated with a *P* value.

2. **The Peto method:** This is for individual and combined odds ratios.

Methods to test for heterogeneity

Forest plot: This provides visual evidence of heterogeneity if present. Heterogeneity is indicated if the confidence intervals of a study do not overlap with any of the confidence intervals of the other studies.

Chi-squared statistic: The Chi-squared test tests the null hypothesis that variables estimated from two or more independent samples are the same and that any difference is due to chance alone. Quoted in a meta-analysis, the Chi-squared statistic indicates whether there is any variation between the results displayed over and above what would be expected by chance. A low *P* value (or a large Chi-squared statistic relative to its degree of freedom) may provide evidence of heterogeneity. The **Mantel–Haenszel test** can be used to calculate the Chi-squared distribution.

Z statistic: If a Z statistic is quoted, this should be associated with a *P* value or confidence intervals. If $Z > 2.2$, the null hypothesis can be rejected – that is, there is heterogeneity present.

Galbraith plot: A Galbraith plot is useful when the number of studies is small.

It is a graph with 1/SE on the *x* axis and the *Z* statistic on the *y* axis. The summary effect line goes through the middle. Heterogeneity is indicated by studies lying a certain number of standard deviations above or below this summary effect line.

Some methods aim to identify homogeneity and as a result can be used to **eliminate heterogeneity**. For example:

- **L'Abbé plot:** This plots on the *x* axis the percentage with successful outcome in the control group, and on the *y* axis the percentage of successful outcome in the experimental group. A diagonal line is drawn between the two axes and above the line represents effective treatment; below the line is ineffective treatment. The more compact the distribution of the points on the graph, the more likely that homogeneity is present and the less likely that heterogeneity is present.

- **Cochran's Q statistic:** Cochran's Q statistic is computed from replicated measurements data with binary responses.

In summary ...

If no heterogeneity is found:

- you can perform a meta-analysis and generate a common summary effect measure, and

- decide on what data to combine. Examples of measures that can be combined include:
  - risk ratio
  - odds ratio
  - risk difference
  - effect size (*Z* statistic, standardised mean difference)
  - *P* values
  - correlation coefficient
  - sensitivity and specificity of a diagnostic test.

If significant heterogeneity is found:

- you can decide not to combine the data, and

- find out what factors might explain it, using one of these approaches:
  - graphical methods
  - meta-regression
  - sensitivity analysis
  - subgroup analysis.

Meta-regression analysis

Meta-regression is a method that can be used to try to adjust for heterogeneity in a meta-analysis. It can test to see whether there is evidence of different effects in different subgroups of trials. For example, you can use meta-regression to test whether treatment effects are greater in studies of low quality than in studies of high quality.

Meta-regression analysis aims to relate the size of a treatment effect to factors within a study, rather than just obtaining one summary effect across all the trials. For example, the use of statins to lower cholesterol levels may be investigated by a series of trials. A meta-analysis of these trials may produce a summary-effect size across all the trials. A meta-regression analysis will provide information on the role of statin dosage and its effect on lowering cholesterol levels, helping to explain any heterogeneity of treatment effect between the studies present in the meta-analysis. Meta-regression is most useful when there is high variability in the factor being examined.

Sensitivity analysis

Sensitivity analysis assesses how sensitive the results of the analysis are to changes in the way it was done. It allows researchers to see if the results would change significantly if key decisions or underlying assumptions in the set-up and methodology of the trial were changed. If the results are not significantly changed during sensitivity analyses, the researchers can be more confident of the results. If the results do change such that the conclusions drawn will also differ, researchers need to discuss these factors.

Subgroup analysis

Data dredging is a common phenomenon of studies, and sometimes this can lead to researchers testing for everything and then only reporting the significant results.

Performing many subgroup analyses has the effect of greatly increasing the chance that at least one of these comparisons will be statistically significant, even if there is no real difference. For example, where several factors may influence outcome (eg, sex, age, race, smoking status) the risk of false-positive results is high. As a result, conclusions can be misleading. Deciding on subgroups after the results are available can also lead to bias.

Multiple-hypothesis testing on the same set of results should be avoided. Subgroup analyses should be restricted to a minimum and, if possible, subgroup analyses should be pre-specified in the methodology whenever possible. Any analyses suggested by the data should be acknowledged as exploratory for generating hypotheses and not testing them.

PUBLICATION BIAS

Reporting bias is the term applied to a group of related biases that can lead to over-representation of significant or positive studies in systematic reviews. Types of reporting bias include time-lag bias, language bias, citation bias, funding bias, outcome variable selection bias, developed country bias, publication bias and multiple publication bias.

Publication bias

Studies with positive findings are more likely to be submitted and published than studies with negative findings. As a result, smaller studies with negative findings tend to be omitted from meta-analyses, leading to a positive bias in the overall estimate. These positive studies are also more likely to be published in English and more likely to be cited by other authors.

If the results of these small studies differ systematically from those that are included in the systematic review, their exclusion means that the overall results are misleading. The over-representation of positive studies in systematic reviews may mean that the results are biased toward a positive result.

There are several methods available to identify publication bias, including **funnel plots**, the **Galbraith plot** (possible publication bias is indicated by a positive intercept for the regression line, which should pass through the origin), and tests such as the **Egger test** and **Rosenthal's Fail-safe N**.

Funnel plots

Funnel plots are scatter plots of treatment effects estimated from individual studies (on the x axis) and some measure of study size on the y axis. The shape of the funnel is dependent on what is plotted on the y axis (**Figure 34**).

The variables on the y axis may include any of the following:

- standard error
- precision (1/standard error)
- sample size
- 1/sample size
- log(sample size)
- log(1/sample size)

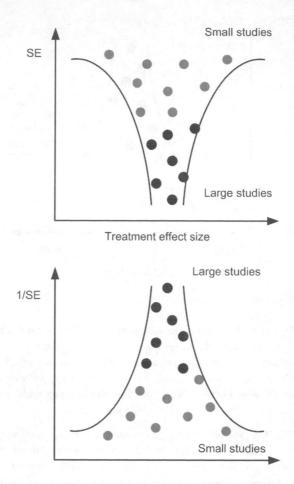

Figure 34: The shape of the funnel plot is dependent on what is plotted on the y axis

Each point on the graph represents one of the studies. Precision in estimating the underlying treatment effect increases as a study's sample size increases. This means that effect estimates from small studies scatter more widely at the open end (widest part) of the funnel. Larger studies have greater precision and provide more similar measures of effect that are nearer to the true effect, and these will lie on the narrow end of the funnel.

Asymmetry of funnel plots
In the absence of bias, the plot therefore resembles a symmetric funnel. If there is publication bias, there will be asymmetry of the open / wide end because of the absence of small negative results (**Figure 35**).

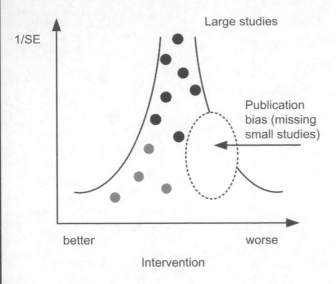

Figure 35: A funnel plot can reveal publication bias

Funnel plots should be seen as a means of examining the effects of small studies – that is, the tendency for the smaller studies in a meta-analysis to show larger treatment effects. The overall estimate of treatment effect from a meta-analysis should be examined closely if there is asymmetry of a funnel plot. Explanations could be publication bias, heterogeneity between trials or even exaggeration of treatment effects in poor-quality small studies.

The **'trim and fill'** method can be used with funnel plots to correct for publication bias. First, the number of 'asymmetric' trials on one side of the funnel is estimated. These trials are then removed, or 'trimmed' from the funnel, leaving a symmetric remainder from which the true centre of the funnel is estimated by standard meta-analysis procedures. The trimmed trials are then replaced and their missing counterparts 'filled': these are mirror images of the trimmed trials with the mirror axis placed at the pooled estimate. This then allows an adjusted overall confidence interval to be calculated.

INTERIM ANALYSIS

Trials may take several months from start to finish. Interim analyses allow researchers to see the results at specific time points before the end of the study. Interim analyses can help to identify flaws in the study design and can help in identifying significant beneficial or harmful effects that may be occurring. This can sometimes result in the study being stopped early for ethical reasons, if it is clear that one group is receiving treatment that is more harmful or less beneficial than another.

There is a potential problem with interim analyses. If multiple analyses are performed, positive findings may arise solely by chance and mislead the researchers. Several group sequential statistical methods are available to adjust for multiple analyses. Their use should be specified in the trial protocol.

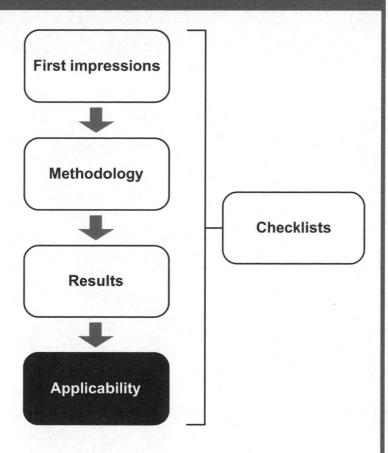

APPLICABILITY

The next stage of critical appraisal is to determine the applicability of the research findings. By this stage you will have decided that the results are significant in some way. Some research findings may be of academic interest only whilst others may potentially help your patients. Providing your patients are demographically and clinically similar to the sample population, it may be worth applying the results to your clinical practice. The following section on checklists gives further pointers to the applicability of results from different types of studies. The decision to go ahead also depends on your expert knowledge, clinical competency to implement the findings and the availability of resources.

Critical appraisal is but one part of evidence-based medicine. The application and monitoring of any changes to your clinical practice are the final steps in modifying your service to an evidence-based model.

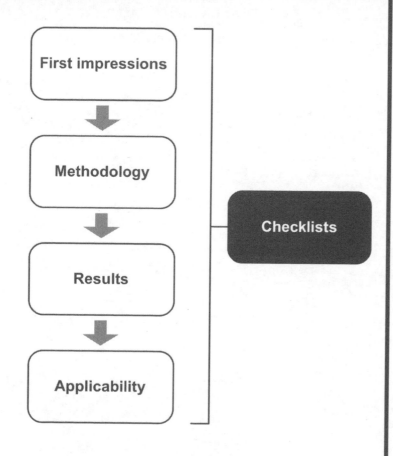

CHECKLISTS

All clinical papers can be understood and critically appraised using the structure that we have described so far. The clinical question and study type are considered before the methodology and results are appraised.

As well as classification of research work by the type of study design used, it can be classified by the subject area of the clinical question. For example, some studies look at aetiological factors; others look at the usefulness of diagnostic tests. Within different clinical areas, there may be specific questions to ask, particularly with regard to the methodology and results. Applicability concerns tend to be the same.

Checklists provide a way to work through the key considerations when critically appraising different study types, by listing the key points in the methodology, reporting of results and applicability. Many institutions have published checklists, but the most highly acclaimed checklists were published in the *Users' guide to medical literature*, published between 1993 and 2000 in the *Journal of the American Medical Association (JAMA)* by the Evidence-Based Medicine Working Group (see 'Further reading' on p. 155 for references). The following chapters in this section give a concise overview of the use of checklists that we use in our clinical practice. To avoid duplication, only new terms and concepts are elaborated on.

AETIOLOGICAL STUDIES

Aetiological studies compare the risk of developing an outcome in one or more groups exposed to one or more risk factors. Study types commonly used included case–control and cohort.

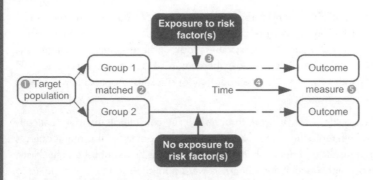

Figure 36: Aetiological studies

METHODOLOGY (NUMBERS RELATE TO FIGURE 36)

1 Was there a clearly defined group of patients?
2 Except for the exposure studied, were the groups similar to each other?
3 Did the exposure precede the onset of the outcome?
4 Was the follow-up of the subjects complete and of sufficient duration?
5 Were exposures and clinical outcomes measured in the same ways in both groups?

RESULTS

Relative risk in a randomised trial or cohort study
Odds ratio in a case–control study
Precision of the estimate of risk – confidence limits
Is there a dose–response gradient?
Does the association make biological sense?

APPLICABILITY

Are your patients similar to the target population?
Are the risk factor(s) similar to those experienced in your population?
What are your patients' risks of the adverse outcome (number needed to harm)?
Should exposure to the risk factor(s) be stopped or minimised?

Table 22 Aetiological studies checklist

DIAGNOSTIC OR SCREENING STUDIES

A diagnostic study compares a new test for diagnosing a condition with the gold-standard method.

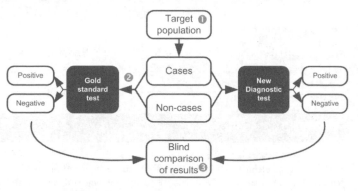

Figure 37: Diagnostic studies

A good test will correctly identify patients with the condition (**true positives**) while minimising the number of patients without the condition who also test positive (**false positives**). Similarly, it will correctly identify patients who do not have the condition (**true negatives**) and minimise the number of patients given negative results when they do have the condition (**false negatives**).

Screening tests look for the early signs of a disease in asymptomatic people so that the disease can be treated before it gets to an advanced stage. The acceptability of false positive and false negative results depends in part on the seriousness of the condition and its treatment. A false-positive result causes unnecessary anxiety for the patient and may lead to expensive, unpleasant or dangerous treatments that are not indicated. A false-negative result may lull a patient into a false sense of security and other symptoms and signs of disease may be ignored.

METHODOLOGY

1　Did the patient sample include an appropriate spectrum of patients to whom the test will be applied?
2　Was the gold standard applied regardless of the diagnostic test result?
3　Was there was an independent and blind comparison with a gold standard of diagnosis?

RESULTS

Sensitivity
Specificity
Positive predictive value
Negative predictive value
Likelihood ratios
Pre-test probability and odds
Post-test probability and odds
Receiver operating curve

APPLICABILITY

Are your patients similar to the target population?
Is it possible to integrate this test into your clinical settings and procedures?
Who will carry out the test in your clinical setting and who will interpret the results?
Will the results of the test affect your management of the patient?
Is the test affordable?

Table 23 Diagnostic or screening studies checklist

Characteristics of the test

The results of the comparison of a diagnostic test with a gold-standard test need to be tabulated in a 2 × 2 table, as shown in **Table 24**. The values of *a*, *b*, *c* and *d* will either be given or can be deduced from other data given in the results section.

		Disease status by gold standard		
		positive	negative	Totals
Disease status by diagnostic test	positive	a	b	a + b
	negative	c	d	c + d
	Totals	a + c	b + d	a + b + c + d

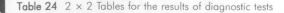

Table 24 2 × 2 Tables for the results of diagnostic tests

There are a number of words and phrases used to describe the characteristics of a diagnostic test (**Table 25**). Each of these values should be calculated. A learning aid to help remember the formulae is shown in **Figure 38**. Clinically, the positive predictive value and negative predictive value are of most use, and may influence the management strategy.

TEST CHARACTERISTICS	DESCRIPTION	FORMULA
Sensitivity (true positive rate)	The proportion of people with the disease who test positive	$\dfrac{a}{a + c}$
Specificity (true negative rate)	The proportion of people without the disease who test negative	$\dfrac{d}{b + d}$
Positive predictive value	The proportion of people scoring positive on the test who will have the disease	$\dfrac{a}{a + b}$
Negative predictive value	The proportion of people scoring negative on the test who will not have the disease	$\dfrac{d}{c + d}$
Likelihood ratio for a positive test result (LR+)	The likelihood that people who test positive will have the disease as opposed to not having the disease	$\dfrac{sensitivity}{1 - specificity}$
Likelihood ratio of a negative result (LR–)	The likelihood that people who test negative will have the disease as opposed to not having the disease	$\dfrac{1 - sensitivity}{specificity}$

Table 25 Diagnostic test characteristics

The sensitivity and specificity of a test can be interpreted using the following statements and aide-memoires:

- **SPin:** When a <u>sp</u>ecific test is used a <u>p</u>ositive test tends to <u>rule in</u> the disorder.
- **SNout:** When a <u>s</u>ensitive test is used, a <u>n</u>egative test tends to <u>rule out</u> the disorder.

There are also a number of risks and odds that can be calculated for the patient (**Table 26**).

PATIENT RISKS & ODDS	DESCRIPTION	FORMULA
Pre-test probability (prevalence)	The probability that an individual will have the disorder before the test	$$\dfrac{a + c}{a + b + c + d}$$
Pre-test odds	The odds that an individual will have the disorder before the test	$$\dfrac{pre\text{-}test\ probability}{1 - pre\text{-}test\ probability}$$
Post-test odds	The odds that an individual will have the disorder after the test	$$pre\text{-}test\ odds \times LR +$$
Post-test probability	The probability that the individual will have the disorder after the test	$$\dfrac{post\text{-}test\ odds}{post\text{-}test\ odds + 1}$$

Table 26 Patient risks and odds

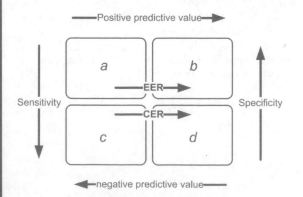

Figure 38: Learning aid for the characteristics of a diagnostic test

Receiver operating curve (ROC)

There is a threshold with any diagnostic test above which a positive result is returned and below which a negative result is returned. During the development of a diagnostic test, this threshold may be varied to assess the trade-off between sensitivity and specificity.

A good diagnostic test would, ideally, be one that has small false-positive and false-negative rates. A bad diagnostic test is one in which the only cut-offs that make the false-positive rate low have a high false-negative rate and vice versa. To find the optimum cut-off point, a **receiver operating curve** is used. This is a graphical representation of the relationship between the false-negative and false-positive rates for each cut-off. The plot shows the false-positive rate (1 – specificity) on the x axis and the true positive rate (sensitivity or 1 – false-negative rate) on the y axis (**Figure 39**).

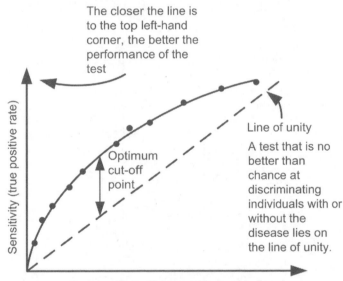

Figure 39: Receiver operating curve

The **area under the curve** represents the probability that the test will correctly identify true-positive and true-negative results. An area of 1 represents a perfect test, whereas an area of 0.5 represents a worthless test.

The closer the curve follows the left-hand border and then the top border of the receiver operating curve space, the more accurate the test; the true-positive rate is high and the false-positive rate is low. This is the point where the area under the curve is the greatest. The best cut-off point is the point at which the vertical distance between that point and the line of unity is the greatest.

Self-assessment exercise 13

1. A new test is developed to test for diabetes mellitus. A gold-standard blood test diagnoses 33 people as diabetic out of a study population of 136. The new test diagnoses 34 people as positive, including two people who were not diagnosed by the gold-standard test.

    a. What are the sensitivity, specificity, positive predictive value and negative predictive value for the test?

    b. What are the likelihood ratios for a positive and negative test result?

    c. What are the pre-test and post-test probabilities and odds?

Treatment studies compare the effects of a new intervention with those of another intervention. A good intervention will improve the outcome compared with previously available interventions. The improvement may be stated in absolute terms, relative terms or by the number needed to treat (NNT).

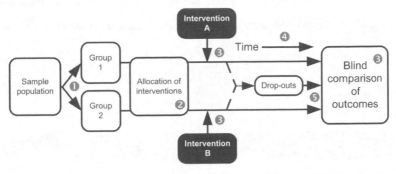

Figure 40: Treatment studies

Was there a clearly focused clinical question and primary hypothesis?
1 Was the randomisation process clearly explained?
Were the groups similar at the start of the study?
2 Was concealed allocation used in the allocation of interventions?
Were the groups treated equally apart from the experimental intervention?
3 Was blinding used effectively?
4 Was follow-up complete and of sufficient duration?
5 Was this an intention-to-treat study?

RESULTS

Control event rate
Experimental event rate
Absolute risk reduction / benefit increase
Relative risk reduction / benefit increase
Numbers needed to treat
Precision of the estimate of treatment effect – confidence limits

APPLICABILITY

Are your patients similar to the target population?
Were all the relevant outcome factors considered?
Will the intervention help your patients?
Are the benefits of the intervention worth the risks and costs?
Have patients' values and preferences been considered?

Table 27 Treatment studies checklist

Translating NNT to your own patient population

The numbers needed to treat calculated in a study may not directly reflect what will happen in a clinical population, where there are many more factors to consider. There are methods available to estimate the NNT for patients in a clinical setting.

Method 1: F

This method estimates the susceptibility to an outcome in your patients not exposed to the treatment, relative to the patients in the trial.

The resulting relative susceptibility is F.

The adjusted NNT for your patient population = NNT/F

Method 2: 1/(PEER × RRR)

The baseline risk that patients like your own have for the outcome of the study (the patient expected event rate, PEER) is estimated:

- from clinical experience
- from studies on prognosis, or
- from your own locally collected data.

This value is then expressed as a fraction and multiplied by the relative risk reduction (RRR) to give a new absolute risk reduction (ARR):

$1/ARR = NNT$ for your patients

Your patients' expected event rate if they received the control treatment:

$1/(PEER \times RRR) = NNT$ for patients like yours

Method 3: Bayes' Theorem

Use a treatment nomogram for Bayes' Theorem.

PROGNOSTIC STUDIES

A prognostic study examines the characteristics of the patient (prognostic factors) that may predict any of the possible outcomes and the likelihood that different outcome events will occur. Outcomes can be positive or negative events. The likelihood of different outcomes occurring can be expressed absolutely, relatively or in the form of a survival curve.

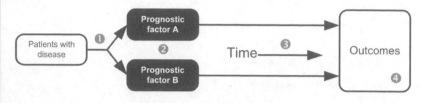

Figure 41: Prognostic studies

METHODOLOGY

1   Was a sample of patients recruited at a common point in the course of the disease?
2   Was there adjustment for important prognostic factors?
3   Was follow-up complete and of sufficient duration?
4   Was there blind assessment of objective outcome criteria?

RESULTS

Absolute risk – eg, 5-year survival rate
Relative risk – eg, risk from a prognostic factor
Survival curves – cumulative events over time
Precision of the prognostic estimates – confidence limits

APPLICABILITY

Are your patients similar to the patients in this study?
Does this study give you a better understanding of the progress of disease and the possible outcomes?
Does this study help you to decide whether to reassure or counsel your patients?

Table 28 Prognostic studies checklist

Survival analysis

Survival analysis studies the time between entry into a study and a subsequent occurrence of an event. Originally such analyses were performed to give information on time to death in fatal conditions, but they can be applied to many outcomes as well as mortality.

Survival analysis is usually applied to data from longitudinal cohort studies. There are, however, problems when analysing data relating to the time between one event and another.

- All times to the event occurring will differ, but it is unlikely that these times will be normally distributed.
- Not all subjects may have entered the study at the same time; there are **unequal observation periods**.
- Some patients may not reach the endpoint by the end of the study. For example, if the event is recovery within 12 months, some patients may not have recovered in the 12-month study period.
- Patients may leave the study early, not experience the event or be lost to follow-up. The data for these individuals are referred to as **censored**.

Both censored observations and unequal observation periods make it difficult to determine the mean survival times, because we do not have all the survival times. As a result, the curve is used to calculate the **median survival time.**

Median survival time

Median survival time is the time from the start of the study that coincides with a 50% probability of survival – that is, the time taken for 50% of the subjects not to have had the event. This value is associated with a P value and 95% confidence intervals.

Kaplan–Meier survival analysis

The Kaplan–Meier survival analysis looks at event rates over the study period, rather than just at a specific time point. It is used to determine survival probabilities and proportions of individuals surviving, enabling the estimation of a cumulative survival probability. The data are presented in life tables and survival curves (**Figure 42**).

The data are first ranked in ascending order over time in life tables. The survival curve is plotted by calculating the proportion of patients who remain alive in the study each time an event occurs, taking into account censored observations. The survival curve will not change at the time of censoring, but only when the next event occurs.

Time is plotted on the x axis, and the proportion of people without the outcome (survivors) at each time point on the y axis. A cumulative curve is achieved with steps at each time an event occurs. Small ticks on the curve indicate the times at which patients are censored.

A survival curve can be used to calculate several parameters:

- the median survival time, which is the time taken until 50% of the population survive
- the survival time, which is the time taken for a certain proportion of the population to survive
- the survival probability at a given time point, which is the probability that an individual will not have developed an endpoint event.
- It can also be used to compare the difference in the proportions surviving in two groups and their confidence intervals, such as when comparing a control population with an experimental population.

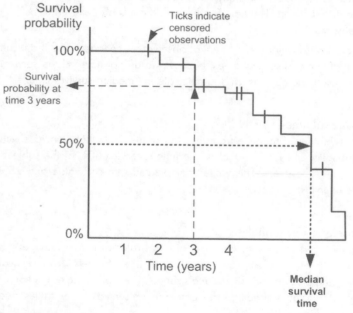

Figure 42: Survival curve

Log rank test

The survival experiences of two populations who may or may not differ according to how they were treated are compared using the **log rank test**. This test uses the Chi-squared distribution. It assumes that the different groups are indifferent – that is, they have the same survival experience. If $P < 0.05$, the results are statistically significant – the null hypothesis of no difference between the groups is rejected.

The log rank test is so called because the data are first ranked and then compared with observations and expected outcome rates in each of the groups (similar to a Chi-squared test). This test cannot take into consideration other variables, in which case a Cox proportional hazard regression analysis is more appropriate.

Proportional Cox regression

This is also known as the **proportional hazards regression analysis** and is the multivariate extension of the log rank test. It is used to assess survival or other time-related events. It explores or adjusts for the effects of other variables.

Hazard is the instantaneous probability of an endpoint event in a study. It measures the degree of increased and decreased risk of a clinical outcome due to a factor, over a period of time and with various durations of follow up.

Proportional Cox regression can be used to produce the hazard ratio, which is a comparison of the hazard values between two groups. Its interpretation is similar to that of odds ratios and risk ratios. If the hazard ratio is >1, the factor increases the risk of death (or specified outcome). If the hazard ratio is <1, the factor decreases the risk. The hazard ratio is complemented by a P value and confidence intervals.

ECONOMIC STUDIES

Resources within the National Health Service are finite. Not every activity can be funded. Economic analyses evaluate the choices in resource allocation by comparing the costs and consequences of different actions. They tend to take a wider perspective on healthcare provision than other types of studies, because they do not just focus on whether one intervention is statistically better than another. They aim to discover which interventions can be used to produce the maximum possible benefits.

Economic analyses can be appraised in much the same way as other types of studies. Much of the debate regarding economic analyses tends to focus on the assumptions made in order to calculate monetary values for the use of resources and the consequent benefits. Such assumptions are based on large amounts of information collected from different sources, including demographic data, epidemiological data, socioeconomic data, and the economic burden of disease.

METHODOLOGY

Is there a full economic comparison of health-care strategies?
Does it identify all other costs and effects?
Were the costs and outcomes properly measured and valued?
Were appropriate allowances made for uncertainties in the analysis?
Are the costs and outcomes related to the baseline risk in the treatment population?

RESULTS

Incremental costs and outcomes of each strategy
Cost minimisation analysis
Cost-effectiveness analysis
Cost–utility analysis
Cost–benefit analysis

APPLICABILITY

Can I use this study in caring for my patients?
Could my patients expect similar outcomes?
Do the costs apply in my own setting?
Are the conclusions unlikely to change with modest changes in costs and outcomes?

Table 29   Economic studies checklist

Cost minimisation analysis

This analysis is used when the interventions being compared produce the same beneficial outcome and the benefit is of the same order of magnitude. The differences in health effects between the different interventions are minimal or not important. The analysis is the most basic form of economic evaluation, because it aims simply to decide the least costly way of achieving the same outcome.

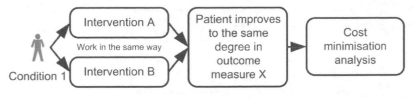

Figure 43: Cost minimisation analysis

Example: the treatment of headache using paracetamol or aspirin.

Cost-effectiveness analysis

In this type of economic analysis, the cost of achieving an effect is compared between interventions. The effect is the same for the alternative interventions, but achieved by different mechanisms and to different degrees. The costs can be expressed in common natural units, for example, cost per unit of health outcome. It can be used to make a comparison of costs and consequences of competing interventions for a given patient group within a given budget.

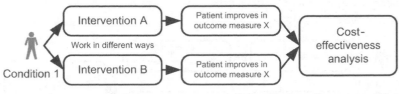

Figure 44: Cost-effectiveness analysis

Example: the treatment of back pain using physiotherapy or surgery.

Cost–utility analysis

A cost–utility analysis is used to make choices between interventions for different conditions in which the units of outcome differ. The interventions produce different consequences in terms of both the quantity and quality of life afterwards, which are expressed as 'utilities'.

The best known utility measure is the '**quality-adjusted life year**' or QALY.

QALY = number of extra years of life obtained ×
the value of the quality of life during those extra years

In terms of the quality of life over 1 year, death is equal to 0 QALYs and 1 year of perfect health is 1 QALY. The competing interventions are compared in terms of cost per utility (cost per QALY).

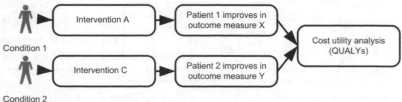

Figure 45: Cost–utility analysis

Example: the treatment of breast cancer using a new drug versus hip replacement surgery.

Cost–benefit analysis

This analysis is used to compare the costs and benefits of different treatments for different patient groups by putting a monetary value on the outcome resulting from each alternative intervention. The results for each intervention are expressed as the ratio of economic benefits to costs or as net economic benefit (ie, benefits minus costs).

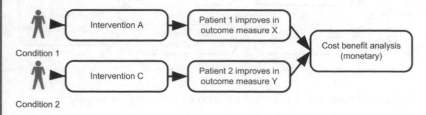

Figure 46: Cost–benefit analysis

Sensitivity analysis

Economic evaluations are models based on assumptions and estimates, and aim to capture and summarise what happens in reality. Sensitivity analysis assists in assessing how robust the conclusions are, considering that there will be a degree of uncertainty about some elements of any economic analysis. It tests the consistency of the results by repeating the comparison between inputs and consequences while varying the assumptions used. The figures are adjusted to account for the full range of possible influences.

A **one-way sensitivity analysis** changes the value of one parameter at a time.

A **multi-way sensitivity analysis** alters two or more parameters simultaneously.

A **probabilistic sensitivity analysis** looks at the effect on the results of an evaluation when the underlying parameters are allowed to vary simultaneously across a range according to predefined distributions. The results it produces are a more realistic estimate of uncertainty.

QUALITATIVE RESEARCH

In contrast to the objective counting and measuring approach of quantitative research, qualitative research concerns itself with the **subjective** measurement of the processes that underlie behavioural patterns. It can investigate meanings, attitudes, beliefs, preferences and behaviours.

As qualitative research helps doctors to understand people and the social and cultural contexts within which they live, there has been an increasing recognition over recent years of the important role such research can play in the formation and development of medical services. Qualitative methods help to bridge the gap between scientific evidence and clinical practice and help doctors to understand the barriers to using evidence-based medicine, and its limitations in informing decisions about treatment.

A checklist approach can be applied to the evaluation of qualitative research (**Table 30**). As with other types of research, a qualitative study should start with a clearly formulated question that addresses a specific clinical problem and that is amenable to investigation by qualitative methods. Examination of the research question takes place in a natural setting where the patient may normally be.

METHODOLOGY

How were the participants chosen?
Was the data collection comprehensive and detailed?
Were the data collected in a way that addresses the research issue?
Is there a relationship between researchers and participants that needs
    consideration?

RESULTS

Was the data analysis sufficiently rigorous?
Were the data analysed appropriately?
Are the results credible and repeatable?
Is there a clear statement of the findings?

APPLICABILITY

Are your patients similar to the patients in this study?
Do the results help you to understand your medical practice and outcomes better?
Does the study help you to understand your relationship with your patients and
    carers better?

Table 30 Qualitative research checklist

Qualitative data sources include participant observation, focus groups, questionnaires, interviews (structured, semi-structured, in-depth), documents, and the researcher's impressions and reactions. The information collected is about how something is experienced, not measured. The quality and depth of information are important.

There are several types of qualitative research methodologies and the **Grounded Theory** is the most widely used. Unlike quantitative methods, the researcher does not begin with a hypothesis and set out to prove it. Instead, using this approach, a theory is developed to comprehensively explain the findings. The development of the theory begins immediately after the data are collected, rather than being deferred until the end of the study, and continues throughout the entire research process. These data are organised and any trends, associations or causal relationships are examined.

The generalisability of qualitative research is usually limited, and these studies tend to be used for hypothesis generation.

HEALTH INFORMATION RESOURCES

Databases

There are many different databases that cover health and medical subject areas and index research and/or high-quality information resources.

MEDLINE is produced by the National Library of Medicine in the United States (http://www.nlm.nih.gov). It is a major source for biomedical information and includes citations to articles from more than 4000 journals. It contains over 12 million citations dating back to the mid-1960s, from international biomedical literature on all aspects of medicine and health care. It contains records of journal articles, bibliographic details of systematic reviews, randomised controlled trials and guidelines. There are many organisations that offer access to MEDLINE, with different ways of searching. The key MEDLINE service is offered by the US National Library of Medicine itself, in their PubMed service (www.pubmed.gov).

Current Index to Nursing and Allied Health Literature (CINAHL) is a nursing and allied health database and covers topics such as health education, physiotherapy, occupational therapy, emergency services, and social services in health care (http://www.cinahl.com). Coverage is from 1982 to the present, and it is updated bi-monthly.

EMBASE is the European equivalent of MEDLINE, the *Excerpta Medica* database, and is published by Elsevier Science (http://www.embase.com). It focuses mainly on drugs and biomedical literature and also covers health policy, drug and alcohol dependence, psychiatry, forensic science and pollution control. It covers more than 3500 journals from 110 countries and includes data from 1974 onwards. The search engine at www.embase.com includes EMBASE and unique MEDLINE records.

MEDLINE, CINAHL and EMBASE are comprehensive, well-established databases and possess sophisticated search facilities. The size of these databases requires that the searcher first defines the search terms and then refines them to reduce the number of results. Although this can be done by limiting to, for example, publication date, language or review articles only, a more valid way of limiting results is to focus on those articles that are more likely to be of a high quality. This is done by using 'filters'.

NHS Economic Evaluations Database (NHS EED) is a database that focuses on economic evaluations of health-care interventions. Economic evaluations are appraised for their quality, strengths and weaknesses. NHS EED is available from the website of the Centre for Reviews and Dissemination (http://www.york.ac.uk/inst/crd/nhsdhp.htm), via the Cochrane Library, via TRIP and via NELH.

Turning Research Into Practice (TRIP) database is a meta-search engine that searches across 61 sites of high-quality information (http://www.tripdatabase.com). Evidence-based publications are searched monthly by experts and indexed fully before being presented in an easy-to-use format with access to full-text articles, medical images and patient leaflets.

Organising Medical Networked Information (OMNI) is a gateway to hand-selected and evaluated Internet resources in Health and Medicine. It was created by a core team based at the University of Nottingham. Access it at http://omni.ac.uk

PsycInfo is an abstract database of psychological literature from the 1800s to the present (http://www.psycinfo.com/psycinfo). It covers more than 2000 titles, of which 98% are peer reviewed.

Ovid HealthSTAR contains citations to the published literature on health services, technology, administration and research. It focuses on both the clinical and non-clinical aspects of health-care delivery.

British Nursing Index (BNI) indexes citations from British and English-language nursing-related journals (www.bniplus.co.uk).

System for Information on Grey Literature in Europe (SIGLE) is a bibliographic database covering non-conventional literature. This database is no longer being updated.

Google Scholar is a new service from the Google search engine (http://scholar.google.com). It provides the ability to search for academic literature located from across the world-wide web, including peer-reviewed papers, theses, books, abstracts and articles, from academic publishers, professional societies, preprint repositories, universities and other scholarly organisations. Google has worked with leading publishers to gain access to material that wouldn't ordinarily be accessible to search engines, because it is locked behind subscription barriers. This allows users of Google Scholar to locate material of interest that would not normally be available to them. Google Scholar even attempts to rank results in order of importance.

Evidence-based medicine journals

Several journals, bulletins and newsletters cover evidence-based medicine and clinical effectiveness. Some evidence-based journals, such as the **ACP Journal Club** (www.acpjc.org) published bimonthly by the American College of Physicians and **Evidence-Based Medicine** (http://ebm.bmjjournals.com), scrutinise articles and summarise the studies in structured abstracts, with a commentary added by a clinical expert. These journals cover reviews and choose articles that meet strict selection criteria. **Best Evidence** is a CD-ROM that contains the full text of *ACP Journal Club* and *Evidence-Based Medicine*.

Other examples of newsletters and bulletins include the **Effective Health Care** bulletins (published until 2004, http://www.york.ac.uk/inst/crd/ehcb.htm) and **Bandolier** (www.ebandolier.com). The latter keeps doctors up to date with literature on the effectiveness of health-care interventions.

Clinical Evidence (http://www.clinicalevidence.com) is a regularly updated guide to best available evidence for effective health care. It is a database of hundreds of clinical questions and answers and is designed to help doctors make evidence-based medicine part of their everyday practice. Topics are selected to cover important clinical conditions seen in primary care or ambulatory settings. There is rigorous peer-review of all material by experts, to ensure that the information is of the highest quality. It is updated and expanded every 6 months and is published jointly by the *British Medical Journal* and the American College of Physicians.

Evidence-Based Medicine Reviews (EBMR) is an electronic information resource that is available both via Ovid Online (http://www.ovid.com) and on CD-ROM. This database combines three evidence-based medicine sources: the *Cochrane Collaboration's Cochrane Database of Systematic Reviews (CDSR)*, the *Database of Abstracts of Reviews of Effectiveness (DARE)*, *ACP Journal Club* and the *Cochrane Central Register of Controlled Trials*.

The Cochrane Library

The *Cochrane Library* (http://www.cochrane.org) is an electronic publication designed to supply high-quality evidence to inform people providing and receiving care, and those responsible for research, teaching, funding and administration at all levels. It is a database of the Cochrane Collaboration, an international network of individuals committed to "preparing, maintaining and promoting the accessibility of systematic reviews of the effects of health care".

It is available via CD-ROM or Internet subscription, and contains about 500 full-text reviews and references to more than 220 000 controlled clinical trials. This is a primary source for information on clinical effectiveness. It contains four databases and several other useful sources of information:

- *Cochrane Database of Systematic Reviews*
- *Database of Abstracts of Reviews of Effectiveness*
- *Cochrane Controlled Trials Register (CCTR)*
- *Cochrane Review Methodology Database*

Development and dissemination of guidelines

The **National Library for Health (NLH)** (http://www.library.nhs.uk/) provides clinicians with access to the best current know-how and knowledge to support health-care-related decisions.

The **National Institute for Clinical Excellence (NICE)** was set up as a Special Health Authority for England and Wales on 1 April 1999. It is part of the NHS and it is responsible for providing national guidance on the promotion of good health and the prevention and treatment of ill health (http://www.nice.org.uk).

The **Scottish Intercollegiate Guidelines Network (SIGN)** was formed in 1993 and its objective is to improve the effectiveness and efficiency of clinical care for patients in Scotland by developing, publishing and disseminating guidelines that identify and promote good clinical practice (http://www.sign.ac.uk).

The **National Guideline Clearinghouse (NGC)** is a USA-based public resource for evidence-based clinical practice (http://www.guideline.gov/).

Other sources of information

Research registers: These are consulting registers of current and recently completed research and give information on other research evidence on a particular topic. For example, the **National Research Register** (http://www.nrr.nhs.uk) has a record of research and development projects either being funded by or of interest to the NHS. **NHS Health Technology Assessment Reports** contain abstracts for the completed reviews from the NHS Health Technology Assessment Programme (http://www.hta.nhsweb.nhs.uk). Health Technology Assessment is the largest single programme of work within the NHS Research and Development Programme. These reports are coordinated at the Wessex Institute for Health Research and Development at the University of Southampton.

Conference proceedings: Papers given at conferences may give important information on new research either in progress or recently completed. Some trials are only ever reported in conference proceedings. Databases such as the **Conference Papers Index** (http://www.csa.com) and **BIOSIS** (http://www.biosis.org) hold records and/or abstracts of some proceedings.

Grey literature: This is material that is not published in the standard book or journal formats. It may include reports, booklets, technical reports, circulars and newsletters, and discussion papers.

Citation searching: This involves using reference lists of articles already retrieved or citation indices to trace other useful studies. The **Science Citation Index** (http://scientific.thomson.com/products/sci) allows searching for references using cited authors' surnames.

Hand searching: Journals can be physically examined for their contents. This is time-consuming, but may be viable when the published data from a topic concentrate around a few key journals.

Searching for information

By adopting a sensible search technique, one can dramatically improve the outcome of a search. You can begin by formulating the research question as 'PICO': patient, intervention, comparator and outcome. This will enable you to perform a more structured search for the relevant information and will indicate where the information needs lie. Keywords, similar words or synonyms should then be identified to search terms on the database.

When you start the search, you want to ensure that the search isn't too narrow – that is, that you get as many papers as possible to look at. This is done by **exploding your search**. This means that you can search for a keyword plus all the associated narrower terms simultaneously. As a result, all articles that have been indexed as narrow terms and that are listed below the broader term are included. If too many results are returned, you can refine the search and get more specific results – **focusing your search**. Filters can be used to increase the effectiveness of the search. Subheadings can be used alongside index terms to narrow the search. Indexers can assign up to 20 Medical Subject Headings (MeSH) keywords to an article. These words can also be weighted by labelling them as major headings. These are then used to represent the main concepts of an article. This can help focus the search even more.

Boolean operators are used to combine together keywords in your search strategy.

AND: This is used to link together different subjects. This is used when you are focusing your search and will therefore retrieve fewer references.

For example, *"diabetes"* AND *"insulin inhalers"* will return items containing both terms.

OR: This is used to broaden your search. You would use OR to combine like subjects or synonyms.

For example, *"diabetes"* OR *"hyperglycaemia"* will return items containing either term.

NOT: This is used to exclude material from a search.

For example, *"diabetes"* NOT *"insipidus"* will return items containing the first item and not the second.

Parentheses (nesting) can be used to clarify relationships between search terms.

For example, *"(diabetes or hyperglycaemia)"* AND *"inhalers"* will return items containing either of the first two terms and the third.

A **truncation** symbol at the end of a word returns any possible endings to that word.

For example, "*cardio**" will return 'cardiology', 'cardiovascular', and 'cardiothoracic'. The truncation symbol varies, including a question mark (?), an asterisk (*) and a plus sign (+).

A **wild card** symbol within a word will return the possible characters that can be substituted.

For example, "*wom#n*" will return 'woman' and 'women'. Common wild card symbols include the hash (#) and the question mark (?).

Thesaurus: This is used in some databases, such as MEDLINE, to help perform more effective searching. It is a controlled vocabulary and is used to index information from different journals. This is done by grouping related concepts under a single preferred term. As a result, all indexers use the same standard terms to describe a subject area, regardless of the term the author has chosen to use. It contains keywords, definitions of those keywords and cross-references between keywords. In health care, the National Library of Medicine use a thesaurus called **Medical Subject Headings (MeSH)**. MeSH contains more than 17 000 terms. Each of these keywords represents a single concept appearing in the medical literature. For most MeSH terms, there will be broader, narrower and related terms to consider for selection. MeSH can also be used by the indexers in putting together entries for Medline databases.

PRESENTING AT A JOURNAL CLUB

Journal clubs are a routine fixture in the academic programmes at teaching hospitals. A successful presentation requires preparation, good presentation skills and clinical relevance for the audience.

Preparation

Different journal clubs take different approaches to the running of the meetings. Some journal clubs are very prescriptive – the clinical paper is already chosen and the doctor has to simply appraise it. Other clubs rely on the doctor to present a paper of his or her choice. Some clubs ask the doctor to search for and appraise a paper related to a clinical question of interest, such as that which might have been raised by a recent case presentation. However the clinical paper is chosen, preparation has to start well in advance of the presentation.

Ideally, you should distribute the clinical paper to the journal club members at least a week in advance. Most articles are available to download as Adobe Acrobat files from the journal websites; this format maintains their original formatting and provides an excellent original for photocopying. However, be aware of copyright restrictions on distribution. An alternative approach is to publicise the link to the article on the World-Wide Web. When you distribute information about your chosen paper, include information on the timing of the journal club and that you will expect everyone to have read the paper before the presentation, which will focus on the critical appraisal of it.

Presentation skills

Nowadays it is not excusable to use anything less than an LCD projector with Microsoft PowerPoint or an equivalent software package for your presentation.

Using PowerPoint

PowerPoint makes it easy to produce great-looking presentations, but its flexibility and ease of use also allow doctors to produce presentations that look anything but professional. Use its template features to give your presentation a consistent and professional appearance. Journal clubs are formal affairs, so stick to a dark background colour for your slides, such as blue or black, with lightly coloured text to keep the presentation sober-looking and to aid readability. Avoid patterned backgrounds and fussy templates, which will distract the audience from your presentation. Use a traditional serif typeface, such as

Times Roman, and avoid typefaces that give an informal impression or try to mimic handwriting.

Slide content

Keep each slide brief and to the point. Every slide should have a title and up to five bullet points, which you will expand on during the presentation. Consider using tables or diagrams to summarise information. Avoid abbreviations and acronyms in your presentation, unless your audience is familiar with them. Make sure you double-check your handwriting and grammar. Pay particular attention to the appropriate use of capital letters and punctuation marks. Avoid fancy slide transitions, animations and sound effects.

Delivering the slide show

Dress smartly for your presentation. Leave your mobile phone or pager with a colleague. Arrive early at the journal club, set up your presentation and make sure all the slides appear as designed – don't expect that the technology will always work.

During the presentation, stand to one side of the screen. Talk clearly to the audience, and not too quickly. Make eye contact with different members of the audience for a few seconds at a time. Wireless remote controls, such as the Logitech Cordless Presenter with its built-in timer and laser pointer, enable you to advance through your slides without having to use the keyboard or stand next to the computer. Using such a device can be a liberating experience.

Slides

The organisation of the slides depends on the subject matter. Below is an example of a slide presentation. Resist the temptation to simply read out an abbreviated form of the research paper – your audience has already read it!

Slide 1	Slide 2
The title of the paper The author(s) of the paper Journal name and date of publication Your name and other details	The clinical question the paper aims to answer The primary hypothesis Comment on the background to this project Comment on originality
Slide 3	Slide 4
The study design – is it appropriate? The target population Inclusion and exclusion criteria The sample population The sample size and power calculations	The randomisation process The blinding process Bias and confounding factors identified

Slide 5	Slide 6
The interventions in both groups The outcome measures Validity and reliability of measurements	Describe the main results

Slide 7	Slide 8
The statistical methods used Intention-to-treat analysis Completeness of follow-up	Were the aims of the study fulfilled? Are the relevant findings justified? Are the conclusions of the paper justified?

Slide 9	Slide 10
What is the impact of the paper? Can the results be generalised to your hospital's populations?	What do you think of the paper? Summarise the good points Summarise the bad points What future work can be done? Any questions?

TAKING PART IN AN AUDIT MEETING

The word audit is guaranteed to divide doctors into two camps. On one side are those doctors who leap at the opportunity to improve the services they offer patients. On the other side are those doctors who detest the idea that they should be taken away from clinical work to engage in what they perceive to be a managerial duty. Whatever the attitude towards audit may be, most doctors find themselves doing audit projects because career progression often depends on having evidence of completed audit projects. Importantly, successful audit outcomes depend on a multidisciplinary team approach to ensure practical and timely interventions to improve services. Doctors not engaging in audit do so at their peril and to the detriment of the service as a whole.

Audit meetings usually take place regularly on a monthly basis. To maintain audience interest and continuity, each audit meeting should have on its agenda a mixture of audit presentations, audit protocols for approval and an opportunity for members of the audience to propose audit titles. A rolling agenda should be kept to ensure that teams present their audit projects at the proposal and protocol stages as well as at the end of the first and second cycles of data collection. Only then will audit projects be completed and make a meaningful difference to service provision. Unfortunately it is all too common to see audit projects abandoned after the first data collection due to apathy, doctors moving to different hospitals or a poor understanding of the audit cycle. Each project should have an audit lead who will see the project through to its conclusion.

It is important to distinguish between audits, surveys and research projects. Far too often surveys of service provision are presented as audits where there is no intention of comparing the findings to a gold standard or repeating the data collection after putting an intervention in place. Other doctors present research projects as a way of sidestepping ethical committees as audit projects do not normally require ethical approval. The chair of the audit meeting needs to keep the meeting focused on audit projects and nothing else.

Below is an example of a slide presentation of an audit protocol. Discussions after such presentations tend to focus on the details of the gold standard of service provision to which the local service will be compared. It is imperative that research is done prior to selecting the gold standard to ensure that it is the gold standard! This may mean seeking out national as well as local guidelines on best practice. In the absence of a recognised gold standard, the team may need to make one up or follow the advice of a key opinion leader.

Slide 1	Slide 2
The title of the audit project The names of the audit lead and participants Date of presentation	A description of the aspect of the service that may need improving

Slide 3	Slide 4
The gold standard for that part of the service	Details of the first cycle of data collection Who will collect the data and when? What data will be collected?

Slide 5	Slide 6
The audit tool in more detail	Date of presentation of first data collection and comparison to the gold standard Any questions?

The audit tool is an instrument that facilitates the data collection which may be done on a retrospective or prospective basis. It is usually a blank form to be filled in with data. The audit tool should be designed to collect only meaningful data and not be over-inclusive. The simpler the audit project, the more likely it is to be completed!

After the first collection of data, the comparison of the local service to the gold standard should be presented at the audit meeting. It is at this point that possible interventions to bring the standard of the local service closer to the gold standard should be discussed with the audience. As far as possible the selected interventions should be pragmatic, likely to succeed and incorporate fail-safe methods.

The completion of the audit cycle requires a final presentation on the second collection of data after the implementation of the agreed interventions. There is however no limit to the number of times any aspect of the service can be re-audited.

Done well, audit projects can lead to health-care environments and procedures that are better suited to the needs of both doctors and patients. It's unlikely that any doctor will complain about that!

WORKING WITH PHARMACEUTICAL REPRESENTATIVES

Doctors differ in their attitudes towards the pharmaceutical industry.

Without a doubt, pharmaceutical companies have revolutionised the practice of medicine. They have invested tremendous amounts in research activity to bring products to the market place that benefit our patients. Without their financial clout, many products would simply never have been in a position to be licensed.

The reputation of some pharmaceutical companies has been tarnished in recent years, however, because of the conflict between their research and marketing departments. The companies exist, after all, to sell products and generate profits. However, as doctors, we should be able to focus our attention on the research work, so that we can decide whether or not our clinical practice can be improved.

The company representative role has evolved over the years in recognition of the changes in the NHS and the acceptance of an evidence-based approach to treatments. In addition to representatives who focus purely on sales either in primary care or in secondary care, there are those who work on NHS issues with Primary Care Trusts and, in some companies, others that work with outcomes research. Different representatives' objectives will not be the same! An understanding of the roles and responsibilities of pharmaceutical representatives will enable you to maximise the benefits of meeting with them regularly.

The sales representative dissected

Before meeting with you, a pharmaceutical sales representative will know a lot about you. Information about your prescribing habits will have been gleaned from data on dispensed prescriptions. The representative wants to meet you because you are in a position to increase the sales of their company's products. This may be accomplished by more prescriptions, advocating the use of their products to other prescribers, or because you are involved in research that could be favourable to their products.

After the usual greetings and niceties, the focus of the discussion will move to your prescribing habits. The representative wants to gain an insight into how you make decisions about prescribing issues. This involves asking questions about the types of patients you see, the products you prescribe, the reasons for your choice of first-line medications and your experiences and prejudices against alternative approaches.

The representative will assess your needs in terms of identifying groups of patients in which your outcomes can be improved. They will talk about their company's products and show you evidence of the benefits of prescribing these products for your patients. Sales aids, PowerPoint presentations, promotional literature and clinical papers will magically appear from black briefcases. The effect can be overwhelming, as you are blinded by volumes of impressive data. The representative finishes off the presentation and questioning and asks for some commitment in terms of trying the company's product.

The doctor's viewpoint

Being a passive observer in a meeting with a sales representative is not good use of your time. The representative is usually very knowledgeable about his specialist field and is the potential source of a lot of useful information. You will have your own needs in terms of information you need to be a better doctor, and by identifying these needs to the representative, you can both be in a win–win situation.

There are general questions you can ask to update your knowledge base:

- What is the latest research the company is doing?
- Are there any impending licence changes or new launches?
- Are there any forthcoming NHS initiatives that you should be aware of?
- Which guidelines are in vogue, and who are the key opinion leaders?

If the representative is selling a product to you, you need to focus the discussion on information that will help you to decide whether or not to prescribe the product. Questions you may ask about the data presented can include the following:

- Are these efficacy data or effectiveness data?
- Is the sample population similar to your own?
- What were the inclusion and exclusion criteria?
- What is the comparative treatment? Is it a placebo or is it a head-to-head trial?
- Do the doses used in the study reflect everyday clinical practice?
- What is the absolute risk reduction with the new treatment?
- What is the number needed to treat?
- Are the results statistically significant or clinically significant?
- In which situations should you not prescribe the new treatment?
- Are there any safety data you need to be aware of?

- Why should you not prescribe a competitor product?
- Is this a cost-effective intervention?
- Are there any post-marketing studies in progress?
- Has the drug been through the Drugs and Therapeutics Committee, or has a pharmaceutical advisor been presented with the data?

If you are presented with any graphs, put your analytical skills to the test by looking for marketing tricks in the presentation of data. Examples include the magnification of the *y* axis to exaggerate differences in comparative results, and the poor labelling of the *x* axis to hide the short duration of the trial.

Sources of information

Promotional material
The representative can give you approved promotional materials that list product features and benefits. Sales aids help convey important information, such as data on efficacy, safety, tolerability, compliance, comparative data with competitors, health-economic data, the summary of product characteristics and the price.

Clinical papers
Clinical papers provide you with the original data on which promotional material is based. If you prefer to look at the clinical papers, ask the representative to go through the relevant papers or, alternatively, ask for copies to be sent to you. Once you have the paper, you will want to appraise it critically yourself and then arrange to meet with the representative to discuss any issues or questions that you may have. An experienced representative will be able to critique the paper as they use it to sell to you, and point out key important details.

Key opinion leaders
You may want to know the opinion of specialists in a field before you prescribe a certain drug. Ask your representative about key opinion leaders and whether they can arrange for you to meet with these people or hear them speak at an appropriate scientific meeting. Alternatively, ask to set up a round-table meeting with you and your colleagues so that you can have an open discussion with the expert about the product and how it would benefit your patients. If you would like to be an advocate for the product, then tell the representative to arrange meetings for you to discuss this with your colleagues.

Data on file

If there is information presented that you are interested in but has not yet been published, it is usually referenced as 'data on file'. If you would like to see these data, you can request the information and the representative will contact their medical department, who will send this on to you.

Off-licence data

If you have queries that are off-licence, you should let the representative know. They will contact their medical department, and either someone from that department will come and see you or they will send you the requested information. The representative is not allowed to discuss off-licence information.

FURTHER READING

JAMA series

1. Guyatt GH, Sackett DL, Cook DJ, for the Evidence-Based Medicine Working Group. Users' guides to the medical literature. II. How to use an article about therapy or prevention. A. Are the results of the study valid? *Journal of the American Medical Association* 1993, 270, 2598–601.

2. Guyatt GH, Sackett DL, Cook DJ, for the Evidence-Based Medicine Working Group. Users' guides to the medical literature. II. How to use an article about therapy or prevention. B. What were the results and will they help me in caring for my patients? *Journal of the American Medical Association* 1994, 271, 59–63.

3. Jaeschke R, Guyatt G, Sackett DL. Users' guides to the medical literature. III. How to use an article about a diagnostic test. A. Are the results of the study valid? *Journal of the American Medical Association* 1994, 271, 389–91.

4. Jaeschke R, Gordon H, Guyatt G, Sackett DL, for the Evidence-Based Medicine Working Group. Users' guides to the medical literature. III. How to use an article about a diagnostic test. B. What are the results and will they help me in caring for my patients? *Journal of the American Medical Association* 1994, 271, 703–7.

5. Levine M, Walter S, Lee H, Haines T, Holbrook A, Moyer V, for the Evidence-Based Medicine Working Group. Users' guides to the medical literature. IV. How to use an article about harm. *Journal of the American Medical Association* 1994, 271, 1615–19.

6. Laupacis A, Wells G, Richardson S, Tugwell P, for the Evidence-Based Medicine Working Group. Users' guides to the medical literature. V. How to use an article about prognosis. *Journal of the American Medical Association* 1994, 272, 234–7.

7. Oxman AD, Cook DJ, Guyatt GH, for the Evidence-Based Medicine Working Group. Users' guides to the medical literature. VI. How to use an overview. Evidence-Based Medicine Working Group. *Journal of the American Medical Association* 1994, 272, 1367–71.

8.   Drummond MF, Richardson WS, O'Brien BJ, Levine M, Heyland D,
      for the Evidence-Based Medicine Working Group. Users' guides to
      the medical literature. XIII. How to use an article on economic
      analysis of clinical practice. A. Are the results of the study valid?
      Evidence-Based Medicine Working Group. *Journal of the American
      Medical Association* 1997, 277, 1552–7.

9.   O'Brien BJ, Heyland D, Richardson WS, Levine M, Drummond MF,
      for the Evidence-Based Medicine Working Group. Users' guides to
      the medical literature. XIII. How to use an article on economic
      analysis of clinical practice. B. What are the results and will they
      help me in caring for my patients? Evidence-Based Medicine
      Working Group *Journal of the American Medical Association* 1997,
      277, 1802–6. Published erratum appears in JAMA 1997, 278,
      1064.

10.   Barratt A, Irwig L, Glasziou P, Cumming RG, Raffle A, Hicks N, for
      the Evidence-Based Medicine Working Group. Users' guide to
      medical literature. XVII. How to use guidelines and
      recommendations about screening. *Journal of the American Medical
      Association* 1999, 281, 2029–34.

11.   Giacomini MK, Cook DJ, for the Evidence-Based Medicine Working
      Group. Users' guides to the medical literature. XXIII. Qualitative
      research in health care. A. Are the results of the study valid? *Journal
      of the American Medical Association* 2000, 284, 357–62.

12.   Giacomini MK, Cook DJ, for the Evidence-Based Medicine Working
      Group. Users' guides to the medical literature. XXIII. Qualitative
      research in health care. B. What are the results and how do they
      help me care for my patients? *Journal of the American Medical
      Association* 2000, 284, 478–82.

How to read a paper

A readable and practical series, originally published in the *British Medical Journal*.

1. Greenhalgh T. How to read a paper: the Medline database. *British Medical Journal* 1997, 315, 180–3.

2. Greenhalgh T. How to read a paper: getting your bearings (deciding what the paper is about). *British Medical Journal* 1997, 315, 243–6.

3. Greenhalgh T. How to read a paper: assessing the methodological quality of published papers. *British Medical Journal* 1997, 315, 305–8.

4. Greenhalgh T. How to read a paper: statistics for the non-statistician. I: Different types of data need different statistical tests. *British Medical Journal* 1997, 315, 364–6.

5. Greenhalgh T. How to read a paper: statistics for the non-statistician. II: "Significant" relations and their pitfalls. *British Medical Journal* 1997, 315, 422–5.

6. Greenhalgh T. How to read a paper: papers that report drug trials. *British Medical Journal* 1997, 315, 480–3.

7. Greenhalgh T. How to read a paper: papers that report diagnostic or screening tests. *British Medical Journal* 1997, 315, 540–3.

8. Greenhalgh T. How to read a paper: papers that tell you what things cost (economic analyses). *British Medical Journal* 1997, 315, 596–9.

9. Greenhalgh T. How to read a paper: papers that summarise other papers (systematic reviews and meta-analyses). *British Medical Journal* 1997, 315, 672–5.

10. Greenhalgh T. How to read a paper: papers that go beyond numbers (qualitative research). *British Medical Journal* 1997, 315, 740–3.

Other useful online resources

The **Critical Appraisal Skills Programme (CASP)** is part of the Public Health Resource Unit based at Oxford (http://www.phru.nhs.uk/casp/casp.htm). CASP runs training workshops on critical appraisal skills. This site also contains some of their checklists for appraising research.

The **Evidence-Based Medicine Toolkit** is hosted by the University of Alberta (http://www.med.ualberta.ca/ebm/ebm.htm). It is an online 'box' of handy tools to help you find, appraise and apply in practice, evidence-based research.

Levels of Evidence and Grades of Recommendation is a ranking system used to rank various study designs in order of evidence-based merit (http://www.cebm.net/levels_of_evidence.asp). Systematic reviews / meta-analyses and well-conducted randomised controlled trials are usually seen as the best form of 'evidence', with research based on the outcome of a case series placed somewhere near the bottom.

The Trent Research and Development Support Unit Research Information Access Gateway (TRIAGE) is a very good list of links to critical appraisal resources compiled by the School of Health and Related Research (ScHARR) at Sheffield (http://www.trentrdsu.org.uk/triage.html). The TRIAGE site provides links to teaching materials, tutorials and articles related to all areas of health research and evidence-based medicine.

ANSWERS TO SELF-ASSESSMENT EXERCISES

Self-assessment exercise 1

1. Case–control study

2. Cohort study

3. Audit

4. Randomised controlled trial

5. Qualitative study

6. Economic analysis.

Self-assessment exercise 2

1. All your patients are given the gold-standard test for meningitis – lumbar puncture. They are also given the blood test that you have developed. The results from the new test are compared with the gold-standard test.

2. Your patients will be randomly allocated to one of two groups. One group will receive the new treatment. The other group will receive either a placebo treatment or a pre-existing treatment. After a period of time, the results of the two interventions will be compared.

3. You may choose a case–control study, looking at the risk factors that patients with schizophrenia have been exposed to in the past. Alternatively, you may choose a cohort study design, following up people who smoke cannabis to see if they develop schizophrenia

4. A cohort study of people with and without frozen shoulder are followed up to see if they return to work. Alternatively, one could look at people working and not working and see if any of them have been diagnosed with frozen shoulder.

Self-assessment exercise 3

1. A crossover design requires fewer subjects than a randomised controlled trial because the subjects are their own controls, so they are perfectly matched. However, crossover designs suffer with order effects, historical controls and carry-over effects.

2. Cohort studies observe people who have been exposed to a risk factor to see if they develop an outcome. Case–control studies look at people who already have the outcome and investigate what risk factors they have been exposed to in the past. For investigating rare exposures, cohort studies are better. For investigating rare outcomes, case–control studies are preferred.

3. As a clinician, you should only audit aspects of the service in which you are involved. For example, if you are a doctor in a hospital setting, you should not audit aspects of service provision in a primary care setting. If you did want to audit something that is related to your service but is managed in the primary care setting, it would be acceptable to do a joint project with one of your primary care colleagues.

Self-assessment exercise 4

Any other significant findings should be regarded as exploratory only, and perhaps give you ideas for further research projects.

Self-assessment exercise 5

1. Selection bias: Patients who have suffered cerebrovascular accidents may no longer live at home, or they may be unable to answer the phone.

2. Observation bias: Teenagers may be reluctant to answer questions about drug misuse if questioned by a figure of authority.

3. Selection bias: There will be a concentration of such cases on the ward, resulting in a stronger association than perhaps there is in reality.

4. Observation bias: In the glow of motherhood or after the trauma of childbirth, women may not accurately recall the pain of delivery and the interventions used.

Self-assessment exercise 6
1.
    a. Smoking cigarettes

    b. Fair skin

    c. Smoking

    d. Poverty.

2.   Inclusion criteria include:

- Adult age group 18–65 years (licence restrictions; criteria for admission to adult wards)
- Diagnosed with schizoaffective disorder
- Hospital inpatient.

Exclusion criteria include:

- Already taking risperidone
- Treatment failure with risperidone in the past [ethical consideration]
- Co-morbid medical and psychiatric conditions
- Coexisting alcohol / drug misuse
- Unable to give informed consent.

Exercise 7
1.   Annual incidence rate of lung cancer in the exposed group

    = 4 cases in 100 men in 10 years

    = 0.4 cases in 100 men in 1 year

    = 0.4% annual incidence rate.

Annual incidence rate in unexposed group

    = 1 case in 100 men in 10 years

    = 0.1 case in 100 men in 1 year

    = 0.1% annual incidence rate.

Overall incidence rate

    = 5 cases in 200 men in 10 years

    = 0.5 cases in 200 men in 1 year

    = 0.25 cases in 100 men in 1 year

    = 0.25% annual incidence rate.

2.   90 babies delivered every month

    = 1080 babies delivered every year

    1 in 2500 babies affected by cystic fibrosis, ie, 0.04%

    0.04% of 1080 = 0.432 babies every year = about 4 babies every 10 years.

3. 1.3 people in every 100 000 die each year from pancreatitis

    = 780 people in every 60 million die each year from pancreatitis

    = 15 people in every 60 million die each week from pancreatitis.

4. 85 000 people with multiple sclerosis in a population of 60 million

    = 141 people with multiple sclerosis in a population of 100 000

    prevalence rate = 141 per 100 000.

5. Effects on prevalence

    a. increased
    b. decreased
    c. decreased
    d. decreased.

Exercise 8

1.
    a. nominal / multi-category
    b. nominal / binary
    c. quantitative / continuous
    d. categorical / ordinal
    e. quantitative / continuous
    f. nominal / multi-category
    g. quantitative / continuous
    h. nominal / multi-category
    i. quantitative / continuous
    j. nominal / multi-category
    k. categorical / ordinal.
    l. quantitative/discrete.

Exercise 9

1.   a. mode = 3

        b. frequencies: value 1 (1), value 2 (2), value 3 (3), value 4 (2), value 5 (1)

        c. median = 3

        d. range = 5 − 1 = 4

        e. mean = $\dfrac{1+2+2+3+3+3+4+4+5}{9} = 3$

2.   a. median = 15

        b. range = 100 − 5 = 95

        c. mean = $\dfrac{5+10+15+20+100}{5} = 30$

        d. The median describes the central tendency of this data set better, because it is less affected by outlying values.

3.   a. median = $\dfrac{30+35}{2} = 32.5$

        b. range = 70 − 55 = 65

        c. interquartile range

        i. split data into quarters: 5, 10, 15 | 20, 25, 30 | 35, 40, 45 | 50, 60, 70

        ii. 1st quartile lies between 15 and 20 = 17.5

        iii. 3rd quartile lies between 45 and 50 = 47.5

        iv. interquartile range = 47.5 − 17.5 = 30.

4.   a. mean = $\dfrac{3+13+44+45+51+56+66+75+91+102}{10} = 54.6$

        b. standard deviation = $\sqrt{\dfrac{\sum (x - \bar{x})^2}{n-1}}$

Calculate $(x - \bar{x})^2$ for all the values	$(3 - 54.6)^2 = 2662.56$ $(13 - 54.6)^2 = 1730.56$ $(44 - 54.6)^2 = 112.36$ $(45 - 54.6)^2 = 92.16$ $(51 - 54.6)^2 = 12.96$ $(56 - 54.6)^2 = 1.96$ $(66 - 54.6)^2 = 129.96$ $(75 - 54.6)^2 = 416.16$ $(91 - 54.6)^2 = 1324.96$ $(102 - 54.6)^2 = 2246.76$
Add all the $(x - \bar{x})^2$ values	8730.4
Divide by $n - 1$ ($n = 10$)	$\dfrac{8730.4}{10 - 1} = 970.04$
Standard deviation is the square root of the result	$\sqrt{970.04} = 31.15$

c. 95% of observations will lie two standard deviations on either side of the mean.

mean = 54.6

standard deviation = 31.15

2 standard deviations = 31.15 × 2 = 62.3

range = 54.6 ± 62.3 = –7.7 to 116.9.

Exercise 10

1.   a. mean = 16

            b. median = 17

            c. standard deviation = 3.9

            d. standard error = 1.47.

2.   a. mean = 26

            b. median = 17

            c. standard deviation = 28.8

            d. standard error = 10.88.

Exercise 11

1. Paroxetine is not associated with discontinuation symptoms.

2. Atorvastatin is as effective at lowering cholesterol levels as simvastatin

   or

   Atorvastatin is no more effective than simvastatin at lowering cholesterol levels.

Exercise 12

1. risk $= \dfrac{10}{60} = 0.166 = 16.6\%$

   odds $= \dfrac{10}{50} = 0.2$

2. 5% of 220 = 11

3.

		Lung disease		Totals
		positive	negative	Totals
Exposure to asbestos	positive	20	36	56
	negative	2	42	44
	Totals	22	78	100

$$CER = \frac{2}{44} = 4.5\%$$

$$EER = \frac{20}{56} = 35.7\%$$

Odds in exposed group $= \dfrac{20}{36} = 0.56$

Odds in non-exposed group $= \dfrac{2}{42} = 0.05$

4.

		Fungal nail infection		
		positive	negative	Totals
Given new treatment	positive	21	979	1000
	negative	66	934	1000
	Totals	87	1913	2000

Absolute risk in the treated group (EER) = $\dfrac{21}{1000}$ = 0.021 = 2.1%

Absolute risk in the untreated group (CER) = $\dfrac{66}{1000}$ = 0.066 = 6.6%

Relative risk = $\dfrac{0.021}{0.066}$ = 0.32 = 32% (an improvement)

Relative risk reduction = $\dfrac{0.066 - 0.021}{0.066}$ = 0.68

Absolute risk reduction = 0.066 − 0.021 = 0.045

The number needed to treat = $\dfrac{1}{0.045}$ = 22

5.

		Pain symptoms improved		
		positive	negative	Totals
Given new analgesic	positive	17	4	21
	negative	1	19	20
	Totals	17	24	41

CER = $\dfrac{1}{20}$ = 0.05

EER = $\dfrac{17}{21}$ = 0.81

Odds ratio = $\dfrac{17 \times 19}{4 \times 1}$ = 80.75

6. You can be 95% sure that the true relative risk lies between the values 0.7 and 2.1. Alternatively, you can be 5% sure that the true relative risk is less than 0.7 or greater than 2.1. Note that the range of the relative risk contains the null hypothesis value of 1, therefore the relative risk result is not statistically significant.

Self-assessment exercise 13
1. First draw a 2 × 2 table

		Disease status by gold standard		
		positive	negative	Totals
Disease status by new test	positive	32	2	34
	negative	1	101	102
	Totals	33	103	136

$$\text{Sensitivity} = \frac{32}{33} = 0.97$$

$$\text{Specificity} = \frac{101}{103} = 0.98$$

$$\text{Positive predictive value} = \frac{32}{32 + 2} = 0.94$$

$$\text{Negative predictive value} = \frac{101}{1 + 101} = 0.99$$

$$\text{Likelihood ratio for a positive test result} = \frac{0.97}{1 - 0.98} = 48.5$$

$$\text{Likelihood ratio for a negative test result} = \frac{1 - 0.97}{0.98} = 0.03$$

$$\text{Pre-test probability} = \frac{32 + 1}{32 + 2 + 1 + 101} = 0.24$$

$$\text{Pre-test odds} = \frac{0.24}{1 - 0.24} = 0.31$$

$$\text{Post-test odds} = 0.31 \times 48.5 = 15.03$$

$$\text{Post-test probability} = \frac{15.03}{15.03 + 1} = 0.94$$

A FINAL THOUGHT

It is never an easy task to initiate, plan and complete a research project. It requires dedication, hard work and a willingness to work long hours, which are often unpaid and unrecognised. Few researchers aim deliberately to publish poor-quality research. More often than not, limitations in trial design and conduct are due to a lack of resources, ethical considerations or simply that pragmatic solutions have to be found to enable the research project to take place.

The attainment of critical appraisal skills allows doctors to evaluate the quality of research papers. Such skills should be used, not only to find flaws in clinical papers, but also to comment positively on the good points. Taking a balanced approach will ensure that all research, good and bad, generates ideas for future projects. It is this endless cycle of thinking, questioning and doing that has brought us so far. The journey is far from complete.

In 1676, Isaac Newton wrote to a fellow scientist, acknowledging the work of others in his own research: "If I have seen further, it is by standing on the shoulders of giants."

INDEX